Palgrave Studies in Cyberpsychology

Series Editor
Jens Binder
Nottingham Trent University
Nottingham, UK

Palgrave Studies in Cyberpsychology aims to foster and to chart the scope of research driven by a psychological understanding of the effects of the 'new technology' that is shaping our world after the digital revolution. The series takes an inclusive approach and considers all aspects of human behaviours and experiential states in relation to digital technologies, to the Internet, and to virtual environments. As such, Cyberpsychology reaches out to several neighbouring disciplines, from Human-Computer Interaction to Media and Communication Studies. A core question underpinning the series concerns the actual psychological novelty of new technology. To what extent do we need to expand conventional theories and models to account for cyberpsychological phenomena? At which points is the ubiquitous digitisation of our everyday lives shifting the focus of research questions and research needs? Where do we see implications for our psychological functioning that are likely to outlast shortlived fashions in technology use?

Lewis Goodings • Darren Ellis
Ian Tucker

Understanding Mental Health Apps

An Applied Psychosocial Perspective

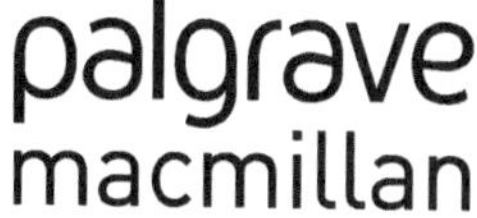

Lewis Goodings
School of Psychology and
Sport Science
Anglia Ruskin University
Cambridge, UK

Darren Ellis
School of Social Sciences
University of the West of England
Bristol, UK

Ian Tucker
School of Psychology
University of East London
London, UK

ISSN 2946-2754 ISSN 2946-2762 (electronic)
Palgrave Studies in Cyberpsychology
ISBN 978-3-031-53910-7 ISBN 978-3-031-53911-4 (eBook)
https://doi.org/10.1007/978-3-031-53911-4

This Palgrave Macmillan imprint is published by the registered company Springer Nature Switzerland AG.
The registered company address is: Gewerbestrasse 11, 6330 Cham, Switzerland

Paper in this product is recyclable.

Acknowledgments

This book is the culmination of a variety of projects exploring the role of apps in our everyday lives, which is an ongoing project and one that has seen us work together for several years. We would like to thank the participants that feature in this book and in the other research projects we have conducted over the years. Without your insight, none of this would be possible. We need to give a special mention to James Ritchie for his guidance in the collection of the Reddit data. Thanks, James.

We feel it's important to acknowledge the people that got us started down this road of applied social psychology and affect: Steve Brown, Paula Reavey, John Cromby, Abi Locke, Paul Stenner, Tony Sampson, and Dave Harper. We are very grateful for all your guidance and kindness.

We would also like to thank current colleagues and friends. Lewis would particularly like to thank Matt Bristow, David Pearson, Nic Gibson, Emma Kaminskiy, and Mick Finlay for their continued support and friendship at ARU.

To Marcia Worrell, who brought joy and laughter to so many, you are gone but not forgotten.

Finally, we would like to thank our families: Beth, Nora, and Edie; Nicola, Lily, Otto, and Arthur; Noah and Isaac. Thanks to you all.

ACKNOWLEDGMENTS

Contents

About the Authors

Lewis Goodings is Senior Lecturer in Psychology at Anglia Ruskin University. His research focuses on the intersections between digital technologies and mental health. His work is dedicated to an applied version of social psychology that focuses on the role of space and place, with an overriding interest on the affective aspects of interaction. He has published in a range of journals on these topics including *New, Media & Society; Social Science Information;* and *Media, Culture & Society.* Lewis has received external funding from the Economic and Social Research Council (ESRC) for a project on the role of peer-support in contemporary digital tools for mental health. He is a member of the Social Justice and Empowerment Research Hub at Anglia Ruskin University.

Darren Ellis is Senior Lecturer in Psychology at the University of the West of England Bristol. He was awarded a PhD in Social Psychology from Loughborough University in 2007. He co-authored *Social Psychology of Emotion* (Sage Publications 2015) and *Emotion in the Digital Age* (Routledge Publications, 2020). Additionally, Darren has co-authored and edited two books: *After Lockdown, Opening Up: Psychosocial Transformation in the Wake of COVID-19* (Springer, 2023) and *Affect and Social Media: Emotion, Mediation, Anxiety and Contagion* (Rowman and Littlefield, 2018). Darren has been interested in representations of emotion, for example, how it is experienced and conceptualized. This has led to research in areas such as surveillance studies, social media, and psychotherapy contexts. Darren is also a practicing psychotherapist.

Ian Tucker is Professor of Health and Social Psychology at the University of East London. His research focuses on mental health, emotion, and affect with a specific focus on how they are shaped through interactions with digital technologies. He has published widely in these areas, including *Emotion in the Digital Age* (Routledge, 2020).

CHAPTER 1

Introducing Mental Health Apps

Abstract Mental health apps (MHapps) are designed to provide digital tools and techniques for self-managing psychological forms of distress (e.g. stress and anxiety). In a psychological context, the power and efficacy of these apps is typically evidenced using clinical methods (e.g. randomized controlled trials). This chapter will describe the benefits and challenges to using these methods and will then examine the advances that can be made by considering an applied psychosocial approach to understanding MHapps. This will explore the ways people negotiate the emotional and affective landscape of these apps, considering how MHapps allow for certain ways of thinking, acting, and feeling. This follows a vital materialist perspective and aims to recognize how the lived material experience of using MHapps shapes (and is shaped) by the intersection of a range of different bodies (both human and non-human) in the unique space of MHapps.

Keywords AI • Affect • Apps • Bodies • Mental health • Psychological health and wellbeing • Vital materialism

L. Goodings et al., *Understanding Mental Health Apps*, Palgrave Studies in Cyberpsychology,
https://doi.org/10.1007/978-3-031-53911-4_1

What Are Mental Health Apps?

Mental health apps (MHapps) are mobile applications that can be downloaded to a smartphone, tablet, or other mobile device (e.g. wearables). These technologies include tools and techniques for attending to psychological health and wellbeing. MHapps represent a new branch of general health apps that are growing in popularity and prioritize supporting mental health issues through the self-management of distress. These apps include a range of activities for engaging with and focusing on different aspects of psychological wellbeing. It is estimated that there are already over 10,000 apps dedicated to mental health (Torous & Roberts, 2017). MHapps emphasize the ability to assist with issues of psychological health on a 24/7 basis, having the technology in the palm of the hand and accessible at the touch of a button (Miller & Polson, 2019). They are a low-cost intervention and are frequently praised for their potential to fill the "gap" in mental health resourcing (Donker et al., 2013; Hollis et al., 2015).

Bakker et al. (2016) argue that the majority of apps are either reflection-focused, education-focused, or goal-focused, with many apps providing direct content or techniques for supporting positive mental health (e.g. meditation). More recently, there has also been a rise in apps which offer a direct link to counseling sessions with a psychological practitioner (e.g. Talkspace, BetterHelp) and apps which make use of the advantages of peer-support (e.g. Kooth, Side by Side). The realm of MHapps can also include social chatbots (e.g. Wysa, Replika, Woebot) in which users receive support through AI-based interactions and communication. MHapps aim to provide a way of supporting an individual with mental health issues, ranging from on-the-spot crisis intervention for someone who needs urgent help, through to people who might just download a mental health app on a whim. In the current app culture, it is likely that most people have at least one app that is of a mental health nature on their tablet or mobile device.

MHapps are developed in the context of a "global mental health crisis" (Torous et al., 2018) and the World Health Organization (WHO) and other institutions champion the use of digital healthcare solutions to respond to this crisis (WHO, 2016). This is particularly significant for young people for whom mental health issues are on the rise (Crane et al., 2019) and where issues of mental health have been amplified by the Covid-19 pandemic in recent years (Creswell, 2023). As MHapps are popular with young people, they have been labeled as a direct response to the "problem" of the mental health crisis (Hollis et al., 2015; Fullagar et al., 2017). In 2022, the Department of Health and Social Care (2022) released a guide for good practice for digital and data-driven health technologies that identifies the desire for the NHS to achieve "widespread digitally-enabled care" as part of their response to these issues. There is a growing recognition of the area of "digital psychiatry" and the increasing use of digital technologies to communicate and interact with patients (Torous et al., 2014). This illustrates how the future of mental health care is likely to continue to harness the power of digital technology and seek to find ways to ensure that technologies, like MHapps, can be integrated into formal mental health provision.

MHapps include a range of psychological techniques for support, with many apps making use of techniques from Cognitive Behavioural Therapy (CBT). Table 1.1 illustrates some examples of popular apps and the use of the psychological techniques that feature in these apps.

MHapps often make use of tools from CBT, particularly for the treatment of mild to moderate symptoms of anxiety or depression (Donker et al., 2013). This could include other variations of CBT such as Dialectical Behavioral Therapy (DBT) or Acceptance and Commitment Therapy (ACT). These are similar approaches that involve guiding awareness toward an understanding and recognition of life challenges and then focusing on these issues, in a non-judgmental way, to identify improvements. Non-CBT MHapps might also include tools for journaling and self-reflection, a variety of tests and scales for tracking mood, or external links to community forums and discussion spaces. The strength of MHapps has been demonstrated with a wide range of populations including parents (Liverpool et al., 2019), employees (Muuraiskangas et al., 2016), and adolescents (Donovan et al., 2016).

Grist et al. (2017) found that MHapps can address the shortfall in face-to-face mental health service provision in the context of adolescents who self-harm. This shows the potential for these technologies to provide instant support to vulnerable and hard-to-reach groups who do not typically access formal healthcare practices (see also Hategan et al., 2019; Srivastava et al., 2020). Furthermore, Ramos and Chavira (2022) claim that apps present a promising approach for some racial and ethnic minorities given the accessibility of technology. However, they also warn about the perils of advocating this approach and further enhancing pervasive mental health disparities if these already disadvantaged groups are unable to make use of these technologies.

Table 1.1 A few examples of MHapps and associated psychological techniques

MHapp	*Intended for*	*Type of App*	*Psychological techniques*	*Device*
Calm	Mood disorder, sleep, stress and anxiety	Mindfulness via videos and stories	Mindfulness, meditation	iOS, Android
Happify: For stress and worry	Chronic pain, mood disorders, stress and anxiety, sleep, PTSD	Symptom tracking/ self-monitoring	CBT, mindfulness, psychoeducation, gratitude	iOS, Android, Web
NOCD	OCD	Direct therapy, community support, OCD information and education	Exposure response prevention treatment, mindfulness	iOS, Android
PTSD coach	Those with experience of PTSD	Symptom tracking/ self-monitoring, assessment, screening	CBT, psychoeducation	iOS, Android
SuperBetter	Chronic pain, PTSD, mood disorders, stress and anxiety	Gamified app to build resistance, self-tracking, self-care	Cognitive training, gratitude	iOS, Android, Web
Headspace	Stress and anxiety, mood disorders, sleep	Mindfulness courses and materials, community forum, progress tracking, self-tracking	Mindfulness meditation	iOS, Android, Web
MindDoc	Stress and anxiety, mood disorders	Symptom tracking and communication for a health provider	Online CBT following initial assessment, video-based psychotherapy	iOS, Android
MindShift	Stress and anxiety, specifically for young adults	Information about different types of anxiety, guided relaxation, coping plans	CBT	iOS, Android

(*continued*)

Table 1.1 (continued)

MHapp	*Intended for*	*Type of App*	*Psychological techniques*	*Device*
Feeling good	Stress and anxiety, mood disorders, eating disorders, sleep	Positive mental health program through audio tracks	CBT, mindfulness	iOS, Android, Web
Woebot	Stress and anxiety, mood disorders	AI social chatbot	CBT	iOS, Android
Wysa	Stress and anxiety, mood disorders	AI social chatbot	Cognitive reframing, breathing exercises, connection to a licensed therapist	iOS, Android

Available via https://onemindpsyberguide.org/

The next section will explore one of the reflection-type apps (Headspace) in more detail and will explore how psychological support is delivered through an app. This is not indicative of all apps but is intended to provide an overview of the look and feel of a mental health app, giving information on the ways that people connect with the tools, activities, and support services in an app of this kind. The description of the app will be followed by the psychological evidence for its use, providing insight into the ways that apps of this kind are tried, tested, and evaluated.

Headspace

Headspace is a mindfulness and meditation app that has been downloaded over 65 million times, in 190 countries, with approximately 2 million subscribers worldwide (Kolodziejska & Palinski, 2023). Headspace is one of the most popular mental health apps on the market in the UK and utilizes a range of self-directed meditation and mindfulness techniques. Headspace is one of a small number of mental health apps that is recommended to NHS staff in England and Wales.[1] Headspace claims that the techniques are rooted in Tibetan Buddhist traditions involving eight core techniques including[2]:

- Noting
- Visualization

- Resting awareness
- Focused attention
- Loving kindness
- Reflection
- Body scan
- Skillful comparison

The Headspace app aims to incorporate the above practices into the content in the app. Fundamentally, this takes the form of many hundreds of hours of guided and unguided meditation sessions based on well-established meditation and mindfulness practices. The app is organized via the main 'explore' page from the Headspace app where users can select content based on a desired area of focus, e.g. meditate, sleep, or move. These links provide a variety of videos that can be scrolled through and selected, ranging from short bitesize videos through to longer more in-depth content videos. All videos contain instructions on how to complete an exercise and give information on the benefits and principles of mindfulness techniques. Scientific support for these practices is available in the app and users are encouraged to complete one meditation-based session every day to maximize the benefits of the app. Headspace provides a wealth of meditation exercises that a user can watch and complete, such as managing anxiety or dealing with loss. There is content to help with meditation, sleep, movement, and focus. Much of the content can be downloaded and used offline, and there is an abundance of family-friendly content. Like many other MHapps, Headspace monitors personal usage of the app, and this information is then fed-back to the user via the home screen. Headspace allows the user to track their stress and anxiety via frequent 'check-ins' via the app, which will include completing a short questionnaire on their feelings of stress and anxiety. These measures provide a snapshot of how the user is feeling at that moment. Unlike some other apps, Headspace does not use mood assessment ratings to provide information on the users and instead opts for questionnaires that have been validated in the field of psychology (i.e. the Perceived Stress Scale). Research suggests that Headspace provides a means to overcome traditional barriers to engaging with meditation (Mani, Kavanagh, Hides & Stoyanov, 2015). It has also been found to provide a solution to geographical constraints, social issues, and financial barriers that often permit people from accessing support for mental health issues in general (Miles, Matcham, Strauss & Cavanagh, 2023). In a randomized controlled study, university students reported improvements in a range of mental health outcomes (e.g.

depressive symptoms, college adjustment) when Headspace was compared to a control of generic app users, particularly amongst frequent Headspace users (Flett et al., 2019). Bostock et al. (2019) also found that using Headspace for 8 weeks has the potential to reduce work-related stress and improve perceptions of available social connections and support, which corroborates with the typical impact of mindfulness interventions when delivered face-to-face.

Clinical Evidence and Evaluation of MHapps

Since MHapps like Headspace entered the market, there has been a growing interest in establishing clinical evidence for MHapps, with much research looking to evidence the efficacy of a particular app via clinical methods of research (e.g. randomized controlled trials). Given that large numbers of consumers are using these apps daily, the advantages of being able to recognize these apps as a trusted method for the improvement of mental health conditions could be beneficial for use in a clinical setting. For many researchers, the need to collate this evidence is also due to the lack of clinical research that is used in the design and development of MHapps, and a recognition that these apps should be scientifically tested before being marketed to the general population (Rathbone et al., 2017; Walker & Viaña, 2023). In recent years, the bulk of clinical research into the efficacy of MHapps has been typically based on the management and treatment of mood disorders (Alyami et al., 2017; Eis et al., 2022; Firth et al., 2017: Michalak et al., 2022).

Given the growing number of MHApps available, different ways of clinically evaluating the apps have also appeared. In the US, the American Psychiatric Association (APA) devised the App Evaluation Model in June 2019. This model is hierarchically organized and is presented as a series of questions to be considered when deciding if one should choose to use a particular app, e.g. "does the app appear to do what it claims to do?" The App Evaluation Model is versatile and intended for use to both clients and clinicians. This tool, like many others, bears similarity to the first rating tool of this type—the Mobile Application Rating Scale (MARS). The MARS is not specially focused on MHapps but on more mobile health technologies in general and gives quality indicators in four dimensions: engagement, functionality, aesthetics, and information quality. Stoyanov et al. (2015, p. 6) argues that the MARS provides "simple, objective, reliable, and widely applicable measure of app quality". This model requires the user to rate each of the four dimensions on a five-point Likert scale, the mean scores from each of these dimensions is then taken together to give an overall indicator of the quality of any app. Users can reflect on this information to see if it is the right app for them. The scale also includes a measure of subjective quality of the app, which is largely missing from other models. It also asks questions such as, "would you pay for this app?" and "would you recommend this app to people who might benefit from it?" Again, these scores are intended to give a way of quantifying the use of the app and to provide a way of making decisions, for both clinicians and end-users alike, as to whether to commit to using the app or not.

Reviewing Clinical Evaluations of MHapps

There have been several challenges to using singular clinical research methods to support the evaluation of apps. Firstly, researchers contest the ability for users to implement clinical practices following the advice in the apps (Hendrikoff et al., 2019; Huckvale et al., 2020; Stawarz et al., 2018). For example, it can be difficult to ascertain whether CBT techniques are being used consistently or with minimal attention to formal guidelines for use in an app, questioning the "quality control" of psychological tools in MHapps (see Torous et al., 2019). Indeed, there is no formal guidelines for how the administration of CBT (or any other psychological intervention) should be displayed and produced in an app and the presentation and delivery of these interventions is most likely going to be designed with a marketing potential in mind, as opposed to the best way of organizing the psychological resources for the user. In a systematic study, the use of CBT in a range of apps was compared to the National Institute for Health and Care Excellence (NICE) guidelines for the treatment of depression in adults. Unsurprisingly, there was a shortfall in the application of NICE guidelines in the apps and the researchers urged app developers to consult relevant guidelines and standards when producing apps of this kind (Bowie-DaBreo et al., 2020). Fundamentally, clinical evaluations do not address the administration of psychological tools, and developers are "app-timistic" (Eis et al., 2022) about the ways users are able to self-direct themselves through psychological interventions.

Secondly, only a small number of MHapps have been through the process of collecting clinical data, and as a result, it is difficult to make sense of this data in practice, via meaningful comparisons of the overall suitability of an app. This is a concern for the long-term adoption of apps as there is only a small number of these apps which have clinical information presented in the app. With only a small amount of this research publicly available, the benefits of this data are obscured by the overriding concerns over patient safety, credibility, and usability (Melcher et al., 2022). Tied to this is also the concern that information that is gathered as part of these assessments is being used without an individual's permission or knowledge (Parker et al., 2019).

Thirdly, some question a purely clinical conceptualization of the use of MHapps in which the purpose of the app was to move the user from "broken" to "fixed" (Barker, 2014). This connects with a wider critique of the "medical model" in psychology and questions a linear understanding of mental health distress (Cromby et al., 2013). For many, the decision to download a mental health app is not directly driven by a recognizable issue with their mental health, but rather, it is part of one of the everyday apps that people regularly download and explore as part of typical ecology of apps. These actions are related to the everyday mixing of different technologies and different states of feelings, in a way that it is impossible to say that an app was ever directly responsible for moving mental health from 'unwell' to 'well', for example. This relates to a tendency to focus on MHapps in terms of the *individual* aspects of mental health and somewhat obscure the social aspects of mental health, presenting the user as the origin, source, and solution of mental health distress. Fullagar et al. (2017) argues that these tools of evaluation typically promote the self-management of distress and fail to represent mental health as a complex social issue.

Fourthly, in evaluating MHapps via the App Evaluation Model and other similar tools, there is a tendency to focus on the aspects of app usage that can be objectively measured and defined. As a result, this instills a clinical logic to the general appreciation of apps and obscures the more nuanced and complex areas of MHapp engagement. A clinical appreciation of apps encourages a detached and impersonal view of apps that focuses primarily on the outcomes of using an app. Thus, when considering whether to use a particular app or not, the questions that are of most important are about the scientific grounding of the potential impact of the app, as opposed to thinking about what sort of support that might be encountered when using an app. It also assumes that the different types of MHapps (chatbots vs. meditation apps) can all be understood through the same review process, which given the differences across these apps is unlikely.

Finally, and in a wider discussion of the power of digital data, David Beer argues that digital health data includes a cyclical logic which gives a "*promise* of making us better people, healthier, more efficient, better at connecting" (2019, p. 5 emphasis added). Beer argues that these "promises" obscure the real focus of this process which is to assign value to personal data. Beer is not just commenting on the sorts of evaluation on offer here, but of the ways that digital data produces certain ways of *knowing* that are tied to processes of capitalism and power. As a result, Beer asks the question, "How can we detach ourselves from this in order to see what is really happening?" This is a powerful question and demonstrates the market consumption and proliferation of personal data. To study MHapps, as Beer suggests, we need to "detach" ourselves from this sort of thinking and ask questions about what is really happening in this space.

The following section aims to provide a way of thinking about, as Beer proposes, "what is really happening" in MHapps and introduces a way of theorizing the social and material aspects of MHapp use. This is intended to complement clinical evaluations of MHapps by describing the affective life trajectories that unfold as part of the everyday actions in apps. This builds on recent advances in social science of health that identifies *materialist*, *affective*, and *posthuman* frameworks for studying digital technologies. This focuses on how MHapps are part of a complex socio-materiality in which the technology is embedded in a network of relations that mediates an ever-changing set of affective intensities. As Ellis and Tucker argue, "the digitization of mental health support presents a new materiality in and through which individuals can access services as well as engage in a range of forms of communication" (2020, p. 86). Therefore, the growing use of apps for mental health prompts investigation of the way that affect flows through and is maintained by these spaces.

Affective Approach to Studying MHapps

> Mental health monitoring apps as a broader social phenomenon [are] implicated in the production of posthuman forms of subjectivity, instead of merely as a tool for the treatment of anxiety, depression and mental health. (Williams & Pykett, 2022, p. 2)

This is a useful quote with which to begin the introduction to an affective perspective on studying MHapps, as it acknowledges the need to move beyond seeing MHapps exclusively as an instrument for mental health "treatment", and to start considering MHapps in terms of a wider set of affective forces and practices. This perspective recognizes the complexity of relations in which mental health apps are a part and identifies the subjective and nuanced aspects of using this technology. Studying apps from an affective perspective encourages us to think about *how* people live in concert with these apps and to consider exactly *what* is happening in these apps. Therefore, this aims to develop an understanding of MHapps which is not about their physical design and use, but about how people feel when they are moving through the different objects on the app or making changes to impact their psychological health and wellbeing through an app. The study of affect allows for the exploration of the dynamic between multiple bodies (both human and non-human) and the resulting relations that are constituted in the coming-together of these bodies.

In cultural theory more broadly, affect theory provides a vocabulary for the force or interactional dynamic between different actors in a social-material setting, some seeing this as being similar, and distinct, to the use of the term 'emotion' in psychology (Gregg & Seigworth, 2010; Wetherell, 2012). In a widely accepted definition, following Spinoza and Deleuze, affect relates to the coming-together of different bodies and the subsequent ability to affect or to be affected. That is, what a body can *do* rather than what it is (Fox, 2016). Affect is often described as something that hits and captures us and moves us to connect with other bodies (Clough, 2008). The benefit of this approach is to overcome some long-standing dualisms around internal/external, mind/body, and psychological/social that have plagued psychology and other social sciences for many years. This is of particular interest in the field of digital technology as the individual is routinely displaced as a part of function of this technology, and where this perspective serves to immediately blur notions of interiority, exteriority, individuality, and collectivity (Ellis & Tucker, 2020). Therefore, an affective analysis focuses on the relations that emerge through technology, providing a more expanded understanding of emotion and affect as integral to the way we relate to ourselves as bodies, as well as relate to social and collective life.

Deborah Lupton (2020) describes a "more-than-human" perspective to identify how people can live with and through their data, the sort of which might be found in a MHapp, and how this provides an approach which recognizes the entanglement of human and non-human bodies in "hybrid, unstable and generative ways" (Lupton, 2020, p. 42). Incorporating aspects of affect theory, Lupton argues for a complex entanglement of human and non-human actors, in which, the precise nature of how those actors are assembled forms a network of potential relations through which a person can think, act, and feel. From this perspective, both the human and the material are inextricably linked. Lupton recognizes the intensity and affective forces that are brought-to-life in human-data assemblages, building on concepts from posthumanism and feminist new materialism (e.g. Barad, 2007; Braidotti, 2006; Hayles, 2012). This establishes the role of the material shaping of affective experience and identifies the "distributed and performative nature of agency" (Lupton, 2020, p. 27). Here, agency is not exclusively located within the individual or the environment, but is fully distributed across multiple people, spaces, places, and things. There is a strong focus here on the material shaping of experience (or the "thing-power" as Lupton refers to it) and how people can "feel" about their health when mediated via these digital health technologies (Lupton, 2017).

Vital Materialism

The role of materiality in examining the experience of mental distress is now well-documented (McGrath & Reavey, 2015), particularly in terms of the role of material objects in the production of spaces of mental health (Mol, 2002; Pols, 2012; Tucker, 2011). In adopting this approach to studying MHapps the focus shifts from the clinical, individualization of apps to the "vitalities" of affective bodily performances in the everyday material use of MHapps (see Lupton, 2018, 2019). Lupton and Watson argues that:

> Vital materialism perspectives highlight the relational, dynamic, interwoven, and non-linear dimensions of human/nonhuman worlds. Ways of knowing and learning are based in experiencing the complex more-than-human worlds through and with which humans move. From the vital materialism position, humans are always more-than-human, part of constantly changing assemblages with a variety of heterogeneous actors. These assemblages generate lively forces and vibrancies. (Lupton & Watson, 2022, p. 756)

Recognizing the vital material shaping of an experience requires looking closely at the role of technology in any given assemblage; both in terms of spoken ways that people can discuss the impact of technology on their lives and in terms of unspoken, ineffable aspects of everyday experience. The focus is on the *relations* that are routinely opened-up or shut-down in the ever-changing assemblage of socio-technical bodily arrangements. This calls forth the different ways that an assemblage affords an individual to feel as though they have the capacity and the potential to act in any given setting and, equally, the ways an assemblage embeds a feeling of restricted movement or an inability to make changes.

Lupton (2020) recognizes the influences of Bennett (2010) and Coole (2013) in the origins of the term vital materialism. These scholars emphasize the "thing-power" of human and non-human actors in terms of the affective intensities, forces, and actions that emerge in the specific coming-together of bodies in a network of relations. This is particularly interesting in terms of the potential for action within these relational constructs: What are people able to do? How can they move in space? What things are they not allowed to say or do? In this context, the ability to move and change is not located within the individual, and a vital materialist perspective ascribes to the notion of distributed agency. Meaning that, agency is performed between objects, people, places, and things; it is formed at the moment of moving through space and time, constantly shifting and changing as bodies enter or exit the assemblage. Lupton (2020, p. 11) argues that "when humans come together with apps, they are creating new worlds of movement and place". Opening an MHapp and joining the assemblage of relations therein means activating the agentic properties of that space, and the ability to move, change, and feel within that space emerges from the interactions with the digital material entanglement of relations that are located in those, as Lupton described, "new worlds".

Fullagar et al. (2017) criticizes viewing an app as a representational object through which people can simply access their mental health. Instead, an app should be seen as an assemblage of human and non-human actors that are co-constructed in the ability to affect and be affected. This raises questions such as: How can people view themselves via an app? What do they make of the data in the app, and how do they feel they can act on that information? How do other bodies (such as AI) contribute to and support feelings of mental (ill) health? And fundamentally, how do we understand the role of a wider app ecology in the generation of these feelings?

AI and MHapps

To answer these questions, we propose that this discussion of MHapps needs to not just focus on explicit MHapps like Headspace mentioned above, but also needs to include other digital spaces that are considered to have a mental health benefit, that is, social chatbots. These tools use AI to provide human-like contact for support and many of the features are geared to help people manage everyday stress and anxiety. For example, Wysa uses AI technology to help people manage their mental health in real time by suggesting self-care exercises for mental health support. Wysa endorses tools from CBT and collects other wellness information on the user, e.g. feelings, sentiment, mood, and major life events. The use of Wysa and other chatbots have been found to be shaping the current nature of what digital "recovery" looks like (Meadows et al., 2020). More advanced technologies, such as Replika, involve the creation of a digital social companion that is designed to provide real-time support. Replika is an AI chatbot that involves creating and maintaining a virtual 'friend' who is available to talk to and role-play through a range of issues (e.g. there are dedicated sessions on 'managing difficult emotions' or 'positive thinking'). This technology is not solely designed to offer mental health support as with the other MHapps discussed so far; however, Replika has been found to provide general support with social isolation and loneliness (Laestadius et al., 2022).

Looking at the role of Replika and other chatbot technologies provides a helpful reminder of the wider digital media ecology in which mental health apps reside. All apps need to be considered as being one of several apps that interact with other digital and non-digital technologies, through which affect is assembled and distributed. MHapps are not disconnected from other access points to mental health, and there is a need to constantly consider the interactions with other forms of support. In a study of mental health information searching for LGBTIQ+ young people, Byron (2019) shows that an app could be the equivalent of "Disneyland" but without incorporation into existing practices of information sharing and support practices, it would be rendered useless by the end users of apps. This means that an app could have unparalleled functionality or attest to provide the best possible support for a psychological issue, but without integration in existing social processes, the app would likely have little or no impact given that the social aspects of these apps are one of the main reasons for successful integration into everyday life. Therefore, we need to consider how the wider range of apps (Replika to Headspace) and how these apps "come to matter" (Barad, 2003; Clark & Lupton, 2023).

Data in MHapps

MHapps are sustained through multiple forms of digital data, and there has been a subsequent expansion of what are called Big Data practices in recent years. According to Boyd and Crawford (2012), "big data is less about data that is big than it is about a capacity to search, aggregate and cross-reference large data sets" (2012, p. 663). Some have framed these data as running alongside the practices of the body, as forms of "data bodies" or "data doubles" (Lyon, 2014). This perspective relies on conceptualizing data as inherently tied to an underlying subject and their actions, movements, and transactions, in which this data "make up" the people in the system (Lyon, 2014, p. 6). However, this duplication frames data as always being bound to the individual subject and limited by the actions of the body. However, in following a vital materialist perspective, we accept that data has a *life of its own* and where the interconnected nature of different types of data makes it difficult to extrapolate the role of digital data in one dimension. Hansen (2012) argues that human feelings need to be conceptualized as the product of the relationship between bodies and technics, in which "the body's capacity to act is never simply a property it possesses in isolation; it is always a recursive and constantly modulated function of its embeddedness within a rich texture of sensation" (Hansen, 2012, p. 186). Hansen's work encourages a way of thinking about the role of digital data in contemporary media that gives people the opportunity to be taken outside of their immediate experience to encounter "something that would not otherwise be experientiable" (2012, p. 223). This shows the need to study the way psychological support is mediated through the relations that are enacted in the movement of data and bodies. Our perception of the psychological individual is one that is not limited to the boundary of the body, and is immersed in the complex affective processes that emerge from the relationships entangled in body, data, and environment. MHapps are "datafied" spaces (Sumartojo et al., 2016) that are not tied to an underlying subject.

Key Issues in an Applied Psychosocial Perspective

This book will develop an applied psychosocial perspective to studying MHapps and will build on the literature from a post-humanist, affective, and socio-material perspective. As the opening quote to this section suggests, there is a call for attention to be directed to the affective, technical, and sensory capacities of apps, and, in so doing, this book will provide a social account of the psychological immersion and embodiment in MHapps. The following chapters in this book will each focus on a key aspect of an applied psychosocial approach to studying MHapps. Following this introduction, these issues are:

- How data is mobilized in the everyday affective use of MHapps, with specific reference to the ways that information is presented to the user and how they can "track" their psychological health and wellbeing in the app (Chap. 2).
- How social chatbots function to provide mental health support and the challenges associated with interacting with a Replika following a change to the underlying technical system (Chap. 3).
- How MHapps can be considered as part of an 'expanded' digitally mediated ecology suitable for analysis via an Ecological Momentary Assessment (EMA). This form of analysis can provide a way of exploring the way apps function 'in the field' (Chap. 4).
- How a material perspective can be used to develop an understanding of some of the main issues in MHapps including the presence of atmospheres and algorithms (Chap. 5).

Each chapter will offer both micro and macro perspectives on MHapp usage, ranging from the small, fine-grained details of the everyday use of one function of an app, through to the wider, psychosocial implications for affectivity and app usage. This supports the call for apps to be considered in terms of a wider system of mental health care and to consider the sorts of ways that we live *with* and *through* technology. An applied psychosocial approach to studying MHapps is not limited to a fixed and stable understanding of how people use MHapps to "treat" mental health, like that to be found in a clinical interpretation of MHapps, but rather on the complex, affective and entangled nature of the experience of mental health and how this *collides* with both human and non-human bodies in MHapps.

Notes

1. https://www.england.nhs.uk/supporting-our-nhs-people/support-now/wellbeing-apps/headspace/. Accessed March 2023.
2. https://help.headspace.com/hc/en-us/articles/115011850767-What-are-the-techniques-. Accessed February 2023.

References

Alyami, M., Giri, B., Alyami, H., & Sundram, F. (2017). Social anxiety apps: A systematic review and assessment of app descriptors across mobile store platforms. *Evidence-Based Mental Health, 20*(3), 65–70. https://doi.org/10.1136/eb-2017-102664

Bakker, D., Kazantzis, N., Rickwood, D., & Rickard, N. (2016). Mental health smartphone apps: Review and evidence-based recommendations for future developments. *JMIR Mental Health, 3*(1), e4984.

Barad, K. (2003). Posthumanist performativity: Toward an understanding of how matter comes to matter. *Signs: Journal of Women in Culture and Society, 28*(3), 801–831.

Barad, K. (2007). *Meeting the universe halfway: Quantum physics and the entanglement of matter and meaning*. Duke University Press.

Barker, K. K. (2014). Mindfulness meditation: Do-it-yourself medicalization of every moment. *Social Science & Medicine, 106*(1), 168–176. https://doi.org/10.1016/j.socscimed.2014.01.024

Beer, D. (2019). *The data gaze: Capitalism, power and perception*. Sage Publications.

Bennett, J. (2010). *Vibrant matter: A political ecology of things*. Duke University Press.

Bostock, S., Crosswell, A. D., Prather, A. A., & Steptoe, A. (2019). Mindfulness on-the-go: Effects of a mindfulness meditation app on work stress and well-being. *Journal of Occupational Health Psychology, 24*(1), 127–138. https://doi.org/10.1037/ocp0000118

Bowie-DaBreo, D., Sünram-Lea, S. I., Sas, C., & Iles-Smith, H. (2020). Evaluation of treatment descriptions and alignment with clinical guidance of apps for depression on app stores: Systematic search and content analysis. *JMIR Formative Research, 4*(11), e14988.

Boyd, D., & Crawford, K. (2012). Critical questions for big data: Provocations for a cultural, technological, and scholarly phenomenon. *Information, Communication & Society, 15*(5), 662–679.

Braidotti, R. (2006). Posthuman, all too human: Towards a new process ontology. *Theory, Culture & Society, 23*(7–8), 197–208.

Byron, P. (2019). 'Apps are cool but generally pretty pointless': LGBTIQ+ young people's mental health app ambivalence. *Media International Australia, 171*(1), 51–65.

Clark, M., & Lupton, D. (2023). The materialities and embodiments of mundane software: Exploring how apps come to matter in everyday life. *Online Information Review, 47*(2), 398–413.

Clough, P. T. (2008). The affective turn: Political economy, biomedia and bodies. *Theory, Culture & Society, 25*(1), 1–22.

Coole, D. (2013). Agentic capacities and capacious historical materialism: Thinking with new materialisms in the political sciences. *Millennium, 41*(3), 451–469.

Crane, L., Adams, F., Harper, G., Welch, J., & Pellicano, E. (2019). 'Something needs to change': Mental health experiences of young autistic adults in England. *Autism, 23*(2), 477–493. https://doi.org/10.1177/1362361318757048

Creswell, C. (2023). Editorial Perspective: Rapid responses to understand and address children and young people's mental health in the context of COVID-19. *Journal of Child Psychology and Psychiatry, 64*(1), 209–211. https://doi.org/10.1111/jcpp.13626

Cromby, J., Harper, D., & Reavey, P. (2013). *Psychology, mental health and distress.* Bloomsbury Publishing.

Department of Health and Social Care (2022). *Data saves lives: Reshaping health and social care with data.* https://www.gov.uk/government/publications/data-saves-lives-reshaping-health-and-social-care-with-data/data-saves-lives-reshaping-health-and-social-care-with-data

Donker, T., Petrie, K., Proudfoot, J., Clarke, J., Birch, M., & Christensen, H. (2013). Smartphones for smarter delivery of mental health programs: A systematic review. *Journal of Medical Internet Research, 15*(11), e247. https://doi.org/10.2196/jmir.2791

Donovan, E., Rodgers, R. F., Cousineau, T. M., McGowan, K. M., Luk, S., Yates, K., & Franko, D. L. (2016). Brief report: Feasibility of a mindfulness and self-compassion based mobile intervention for adolescents. *Journal of Adolescence, 53*(1), 217–221. https://doi.org/10.1016/j.adolescence.2016.09.009

Eis, S., Solà-Morales, O., Duarte-Díaz, A., Vidal-Alaball, J., Perestelo-Pérez, L., Robles, N., & Carrion, C. (2022). Mobile applications in mood disorders and mental health: Systematic search in apple app store and Google play store and review of the literature. *International Journal of Environmental Research and Public Health, 19*(4), 2186. https://doi.org/10.3390/ijerph19042186

Ellis, D., & Tucker, I. (2020). *Emotion in the digital age: Technologies, data and psychosocial life.* Routledge.

Firth, J., Torous, J., Nicholas, J., Carney, R., Pratap, A., Rosenbaum, S., & Sarris, J. (2017). The efficacy of smartphone-based mental health interventions for depressive symptoms: A meta-analysis of randomized controlled trials. *World Psychiatry: Official Journal of the World Psychiatric Association (WPA), 16*(3), 287–298. https://doi.org/10.1002/wps.20472

Flett, J. A. M., Hayne, H., Riordan, B. C., Thompson, L. M., & Conner, T. S. (2019). Mobile mindfulness meditation: A randomised controlled trial of the effect of two popular Apps on mental health. *Mindfulness, 10*(5), 863–876. https://doi.org/10.1007/s12671-018-1050-9

Fox, N. J. (2016). Health sociology from post-structuralism to the new materialisms. *Health, 20*(1), 62–74. https://doi.org/10.1177/1363459315615393

Fullagar, S., Rich, E., Francombe-Webb, J., & Maturo, A. (2017). Digital ecologies of youth mental health: Apps, therapeutic publics and pedagogy as affective arrangements. *Social Sciences, 6*(4), 135.

Gregg, M., & Seigworth, G. J. (Eds.). (2010). *The affect theory reader*. Duke University Press.

Grist, R., Porter, J., & Stallard, P. (2017). *Mental health mobile apps for preadolescents and adolescents: A systematic review*. JMIR Publications. https://doi.org/10.2196/jmir.7332

Hansen, M. B. (2012). *Bodies in code: Interfaces with digital media*. Routledge.

Hategan, A., Giroux, C., & Bourgeois, J. A. (2019). Digital technology adoption in psychiatric care: An overview of the contemporary shift from technology to opportunity. *Journal of Technology in Behavioral Science, 4*(3) 171–177. https://doi.org/10.1007/s41347-019-00086-x

Hayles, N. K. (2012). *How we think: Digital media and contemporary technogenesis*. University of Chicago Press.

Hendrikoff, L., Kambeitz-Ilankovic, L., Pryss, R., Senner, F., Falkai, P., Pogarell, O., Hasan, A., & Peters, H. (2019). Prospective acceptance of distinct mobile mental health features in psychiatric patients and mental health professionals. *Journal of Psychiatric Research, 109*, 126–132. https://doi.org/10.1016/j.jpsychires.2018.11.025

Hollis C., Morriss, R., Martin, J., Amani, S., Cotton, R., Denis, M., & Shôn, L. (2015). Technological innovations in mental healthcare: Harnessing the digital revolution. *British Journal of Psychiatry, 206*(4), 263–265. https://doi.org/10.1192/bjp.bp.113.142612

Huckvale, K., Nicholas, J., Torous, J., & Larsen, M. E. (2020). Smartphone apps for the treatment of mental health conditions: Status and considerations. *Current Opinion in Psychology, 36*, 65–70. https://doi.org/10.1016/j.copsyc.2020.04.008

Kolodziejska, M., & Palinski, M. (2023). "Train your mind for a healthy life". The medicalization of mediatized mindfulness in the West. *Current Psychology, 42*(18). https://doi.org/10.1007/s12144-022-02814-8

Laestadius, L., Bishop, A., Gonzalez, M., Illenčík, D., & Campos-Castillo, C. (2022). Too human and not human enough: A grounded theory analysis of mental health harms from emotional dependence on the social chatbot Replika. *New Media & Society*, 146144482211420. https://doi.org/10.1177/14614448221142007

Liverpool, S., Webber, H., Matthews, R., Wolpert, M., & Edbrooke-Childs, J. (2019). A Mobile app to support parents making child mental health decisions: Protocol for a feasibility cluster randomized controlled trial. *JMIR Research Protocols, 8*(8), e14571. https://doi.org/10.2196/14571

Lupton, D. (2017). How does health feel? Towards research on the affective atmospheres of digital health. *Digital Health, 3.* https://doi.org/10.1177/2055207617701276

Lupton, D. (2018). How do data come to matter? Living and becoming with personal data. *Big Data & Society, 5*(2), 2053951718786314.

Lupton, D. (2019). The thing-power of the human-app health assemblage: Thinking with vital materialism. *Social Theory & Health, 17,* 125–139.

Lupton, D. (2020). The sociology of mobile apps. In *The Oxford handbook of digital media sociology* (pp. 197–218). Oxford University Press.

Lupton, D., & Watson, A. (2022). Creations for speculating about digitized automation: Bringing creative writing prompts and vital materialism into the sociology of futures. *Qualitative Inquiry, 28*(7), 754–766.

Lyon, D. (2014). Surveillance, Snowden, and big data: Capacities, consequences, critique. *Big Data & Society, 1*(2), 2053951714541861.

Mani, M., Kavanagh, D. J., Hides, L., & Stoyanov, S. R. (2015). Review and evaluation of mindfulness-based iPhone Apps. *JMIR mHealth and uHealth, 3*(3) e82. https://doi.org/10.2196/mhealth.4328

McGrath, L., & Reavey, P. (2015). Seeking fluid possibility and solid ground: Space and movement in mental health service users' experiences of 'crisis'. *Social Science & Medicine, 1982*(128), 115–125. https://doi.org/10.1016/j.socscimed.2015.01.017

Meadows, R., Hine, C., & Suddaby, E. (2020). Conversational agents and the making of mental health recovery. *Digital Health, 6.* https://doi.org/10.1177/2055207620966170

Melcher, J., Camacho, E., Lagan, S., & Torous, J. (2022). College student engagement with mental health apps: Analysis of barriers to sustained use. *Journal of American College Health: J of ACH, 70*(6), 1819–1825. https://doi.org/10.1080/07448481.2020.1825225

Michalak, E. E., Barnes, S. J., Morton, E., O'Brien, H. L., Murray, G., Hole, R., & Meyer, D. (2022). Supporting self-management and quality of life in bipolar disorder with the PolarUs app (alpha): Protocol for a mixed methods study. *JMIR Research Protocols, 11*(8), e36213. https://doi.org/10.2196/36213

Miles, E., Matcham, F., Strauss, C., & Cavanagh, K. (2023). Making mindfulness meditation a healthy habit abstract. *Mindfulness, 14*(12), 2988–3005. https://doi.org/10.1007/s12671-023-02258-6

Miller, E., & Polson, D. (2019). Apps, avatars, and robots: The future of mental healthcare. *Issues in Mental Health Nursing, 40*(3), 208–214.

Mol, A. (2002). *The body multiple: Ontology in medical practice.* Duke University Press.

Muuraiskangas, S., Harjumaa, M., Kaipainen, K., & Ermes, M. (2016). Process and effects evaluation of a digital mental health intervention targeted at improving occupational well-being: Lessons from an intervention study with failed adoption. *JMIR Mental Health, 3*(2), e13. https://doi.org/10.2196/mental.4465

Parker, L., Halter, V., Karliychuk, T., & Grundy, Q. (2019). How private is your mental health app data? An empirical study of mental health app privacy policies and practices. *International Journal of Law and Psychiatry, 64*, 198–204. https://doi.org/10.1016/j.ijlp.2019.04.002

Pols, J. (2012). *Care at a distance: On the closeness of technology*. Amsterdam University Press.

Ramos, G., & Chavira, D. A. (2022). Use of technology to provide mental health care for racial and ethnic minorities: Evidence, promise, and challenges. *Cognitive and Behavioral Practice, 29*(1), 15–40.

Rathbone, A. L., Clarry, L., & Prescott, J. (2017). Assessing the efficacy of Mobile health apps using the basic principles of cognitive behavioral therapy: Systematic review. *Journal of Medical Internet Research, 19*(11), e399. https://doi.org/10.2196/jmir.8598

Srivastava, K., Chaudhury, S., Dhamija, S., Prakash, J., & Chatterjee, K. (2020). Digital technological interventions in mental health care. *Industrial Psychiatry Journal, 29*(2), 181.

Stawarz, K., Preist, C., Tallon, D., Wiles, N., & Coyle, D. (2018). *User experience of cognitive behavioral therapy apps for depression: An analysis of app functionality and user reviews*. JMIR Publications. https://doi.org/10.2196/10120

Stoyanov, S. R., Hides, L., Kavanagh, D. J., Zelenko, O., Tjondronegoro, D., & Mani, M. (2015). Mobile app rating scale: A new tool for assessing the quality of health Mobile apps. *JMIR mHealth and uHealth, 3*(1), e27. https://doi.org/10.2196/mhealth.3422

Sumartojo, S., Pink, S., Lupton, D., & LaBond, C. H. (2016). The affective intensities of datafied space. *Emotion, Space and Society, 21*, 33–40.

Torous, J., & Roberts, L. W. (2017). Needed innovation in digital health and smartphone applications for mental health: Transparency and trust. *JAMA Psychiatry, 74*(5), 437–438. https://doi.org/10.1001/jamapsychiatry.2017.0262

Torous, J., Keshavan, M., & Gutheil, T. (2014). Promise and perils of digital psychiatry. *Asian Journal of Psychiatry, 10*, 120–122.

Torous, J., Nicholas, J., Larsen, M. E., Firth, J., & Christensen, H. (2018). Clinical review of user engagement with mental health smartphone apps: Evidence, theory and improvements. *BMJ Ment Health, 21*(3), 116–119.

Torous, J., Andersson, G., Bertagnoli, A., Christensen, H., Cuijpers, P., Firth, J., Haim, A., Hsin, H., Hollis, C., Lewis, S., Mohr, D. C., Pratap, A., Roux, S., Sherrill, J., & Arean, P. A. (2019). *Towards a consensus around standards for smartphone apps and digital mental health*. Wiley. https://doi.org/10.1002/wps.20592

Tucker, I. (2011). Somatic concerns of mental health service users: A specific tale of affect. *Distinktion: Scandinavian Journal of Social Theory, 12*(1), 23–35.
Walker, S. L., & Viaña, J. N. (2023). Mindful mindfulness reporting: Media portrayals of scientific evidence for meditation mobile apps. *Public Understanding of Science, 32*(5), 561–579. https://doi.org/10.1177/09636625221147794
Wetherell, M. (2012). Affect and emotion: A new social science understanding. Sage Publications.
Williams, J. E., & Pykett, J. (2022). Mental health monitoring apps for depression and anxiety in children and young people: A scoping review and critical ecological analysis. *Social Science & Medicine*, 297. https://doi.org/10.1016/j.socscimed.2022.114802
World Health Organization. (2016). *Monitoring and evaluating digital health interventions: A practical guide to conducting research and assessment.* Geneva: World Health Organization; 2016. Licence: CC BY-NC-SA 3.0 IGO.

CHAPTER 2

Self-tracking in Mental Health Apps

Abstract In this chapter, we discuss the role of self-tracking in the everyday use of MHapps. Self-tracking is a prominent feature of many MHapps and relates to the multiple and varied ways of *giving a number* to psychological health and then *tracking* changes to this data, in the context of the app. This chapter explores how users of MHapps experience the flow of affective atmospheres in the practices of documenting and tracking their actions. The analysis also explores the encounters with other (non-human) bodies, such as algorithms, that are present at the site of self-tracking. This focuses on the ways the users are able to creatively engage with this spatial and temporal aspects of affective atmospheres in MHapps for possible future action and movement.

Keywords Algorithms • Atmospheres • Feelings • Self-tracking • Psychological health • Vitality

Introduction

Felix Krause (https://howisfelix.today/) is a good example of self-tracking. Felix first launched a website in 2015 (initially called whereisFelix.today) so he could inform his friends and family about the details of his upcoming trips and vacations, making it easy for people to meet up with

L. Goodings et al., *Understanding Mental Health Apps*, Palgrave Studies in Cyberpsychology,
https://doi.org/10.1007/978-3-031-53911-4_2

him. Propelled by the success of tracking this social aspect of his life, Felix began tracking a range of other aspects of his body and associated behaviors including his resting heart rate, the number of vegetables eaten in a day, sleep quality, weight, number of alcoholic drinks consumed, and time spent at his computer. Felix also began collecting information on his current mood and his social life more generally. It is at this point that Felix upgraded his website from 'where is Felix today' to the more accurate '*how* is Felix today'. As Felix argues in a recent TED talk, the data was no longer just about travel plans and social events, it was about "all of me". Felix's website presents data from a variety of digital devices, which enables him to track his life, monitor his body, and share this information with his family and friends. Since 2019, the site has amassed over 400,000 data points, and all the information is presented on the website, making it possible to log-on at any moment and see exactly how Felix is doing, where he is in the world, and a variety of other pieces of information on his life.

Self-tracking is the process of capturing, monitoring, analyzing, and sharing personal data. This concept is frequently linked with the Quantified Self (QS) movement, which emphasizes an appreciation of "self-knowledge through numbers". Self-tracking is not a new process, and people have been found to self-track as early as the eighteenth century (Neff & Nafus, 2016). However, nowadays there are an ever-increasing number of digital opportunities for collecting and recording the body, for example, data can be collected from a variety of methods including biometric sensors via wearable technologies that produce data on heart rate, blood pressure, and sweat rate; devices for recording information on sleep, physical exercise, chronic pain, menstrual cycles, and diet; and ways of measuring internal aspects of the body such as the amount of bacteria in the gut or blood chemistry through digestible sensors. Following the QS movement, data is given a game-like status and there are goals and achievements associated with 'unlocking' a certain level of bio-data capture. Ajana (2018) argues that this constitutes a growing "metric culture" that is driven by self-monitoring of personal data and information. In this chapter, we explore the ways that MHapps make use of self-tracking and the impacts on how people experience tools for mental health support when united with the practices of self-tracking.

MHapps contain multiple ways of recording and capturing information of a psychological nature. To collect this information, an app will typically use a separate measure or scale of a psychological variable. For example, if an app wanted to measure mood, this would need to be established on some form of scale, which can be as simple as a 1–5 scale (1 = low, 5 = high) for recording a mood in that moment. Otherwise, the app could include more sophisticated measures of a psychological construct, such as depression, which would require the use of a validated scale from psychology, e.g. the Patient Health Questionnaire 9 (PHQ-9). MHapps often include opportunities for collecting psychological data before and after completing an exercise in the app. This gives the user opportunities to recognize moments where their psychological health has been improved (or not) by their actions. The data is traditionally shown on the home-screen of the app in an aggregate form and will contain various numerical and visual presentations of the data. The app might also collect information from the app usage itself, for example, Headspace tracks time spent on the app, number of sessions completed, and average duration spent on the app. Other apps, like Calm, track the overall "mindful minutes" (time spent using one of the activities from the app), number of sessions completed, and the longest number of consecutive days of meditation. This information is combined with the self-report data and presented to the user. In the future, this data is also likely to include data from wearable sensors that measure biological signals such as cardiac activity, respiration patterns, and the secretion of stress hormones (Kang & Chai, 2022). In regularly using an app, each user is being informed of their mental health status via the data on the screen, prompting them to make decisions about future possibilities for action (both in and out of the app) based on an appreciation of this data.

Self-monitoring via an app is found to be a powerful tool in increasing emotional self-awareness, providing a way of making sense of previous experiences (Schueller et al., 2021). In an analysis of user reviews, Alqahtani and Orji (2020) identify the importance of being able to track a variety of information as one of the key elements that users liked about using MHapps. Rubanovich et al. (2017) also finds that many people report being drawn to MHapps in the first instance due to the tracking features of the app. Luxton et al. (2011) shows that users can view their information over a given time and this can, without professional intervention, be used to self-diagnose "symptoms" and measure treatment outcomes. Matthews, Murnane and Snyder (2017) looked at the use of self-tracking in relation to the experience of bipolar disorder and found that the information gathered in bipolar-oriented apps was fundamentally organized to provide clinicians with information on mood and medication, as opposed to providing tools and support for the significant challenges associated with bipolar disorder, e.g. coming to terms with diagnosis. As a result, many of the participants in this study had identified alternative ways of tracking their mood and resisted the commercially available clinically oriented apps. As Matthews, Murnane and Snyder (2017, p. 438) argue, "if self-tracking is only considered in the context of standardized rubrics there is a risk of both normative expectations and pressures related to adherence". There is then a need, as outlined in the first chapter, to resist a purely clinical explanation of the everyday uses of apps and explore more socio-material explanations of app usage. Ruckenstein and Pantzar (2015) argue for the need to expand the QS metaphor to explore the everyday "affectual understandings" that are embedded in self-tracking practices.

Thinking critically about the challenges of using of self-tracking in apps, Williams and Pykett (2022) argue that apps place responsibility on the individual to manage and treat their own distress, in which the apps do not typically allow the user much room for uncertainty, meaning that it is easy to be labeled "stressed" or "anxious" via this process. Furthermore, Lupton and Jutel (2015) argue that the quantification of personal data has the potential to "delimit" and "re-order" the ways that bodily signals are reported, understood, interpreted, and treated. Therefore, being able to interact with the practice of identifying symptoms and managing treatments highlights the need for examination of the actual experience of using apps for tracking our psychological health and wellbeing. This chapter will explore the socio-material shaping of the use of MHapps and will seek to investigate a deeper understanding of the social shaping of self-tracking in an everyday context.

A Vital Material Approach to Self-tracking

Lupton (2016a, 2016b, 2017, 2020) has worked extensively with the concept of digital self-tracking to establish the practice of reviewing and processing information as an embodied activity, recognizing the role of human/data assemblages in the processes of making sense of digital data. Lupton (2020) acknowledges that self-tracking can be a response to the need to try and exert control over an unsettling or challenging experience. This is particularly relevant for self-tracking in MHapps as Lupton (2016a) shows how the "lure" of the numbers and the visualization of data transforms the body into both subject and product at the same time, meaning that the self/body is configured through the process of self-tracking, instilling a sense of confidence in the data. As Lupton argues, this makes it easier to then "trust" the numbers as opposed to searching for physical or bodily signals that confirm the data in an app. Fullagar et al. (2017) also argues that this type of app invites "a continual affective investment in the mentally healthy self as an ongoing matter" (p. 7). Therefore, through the practices of self-tracking, people gain insight into their bodies and habits: insights that can "contribute to new forms of embodiment and selfhood" (Lupton, 2020, p. 79). This articulates the lively, performative, and embodied nature of human-data assemblages through which people can develop an understanding of themselves and others via self-tracking.

Self-tracking is a multi-layered experience, operating through the different elements and dimensions. Pink and Fors (2017) note that "self-tracking technologies are involved in the complexities and contingencies of wider environmental configurations with humans, rather than simply being technological objects, which can be studied for their capacity to generate contingent affects or other qualities with humans" (Pink & Fors, 2017, p. 385). This shows the ways self-tracking processes immediately expand beyond the individual and connect with the activities of data and bodies. Lomborg and Frandsen (2016) also argue that self-tracking is a "communicative phenomenon" whereby the act of self-tracking forges a dialogue with not only the self, but also with a wider system and a network of peers. Freeman and Neff (2023) identify the complex relationship between self-tracking in terms of individual, social, and institutional nuances. Therefore, this moves us toward an understanding of the psychological individual that is constituted through the practices of self-tracking, which are always-already embodied via the processes of data and bodies. The self is ***digitally mediated*** in the affective processes of coming-to-know ourselves (and others) as datafied bodies in space.

Self-tracking is also frequently considered in terms of the connections with capitalism and power. Sanders (2017) argues that self-tracking expands "individuals' capacity for self-knowledge and self-care while they serve the convergent interest of biopower and gender retrenchment" (p. 38). Following this perspective, self-tracking serves to normalize contemporary forms of biopower and patriarchy. Shoshana Zuboff (2019) uses the term "surveillance capitalism" to describe the way data is aligned with practices of capital, which are based on extracting data on people through hidden and obscure methods, often without fair compensation or appropriate consent. Meaning that the data which users are continuously providing as they report their experiences of taking part in a mental health exercise in an app, for example, constitutes a form of "dataveillance" that is a powerful commodity in modern society as a way of regulating and governing behavior (van Dijck, 2014). Therefore, any act of self-tracking immediately also connects with big data networks and the distribution of power. Although the discussion of power is not central to the argument in this book, it is important to recognize that the processes are designed to enact capitalist norms and values. Alternatively, this work is on the lively production of data and the experience of the way that affect flows through these spaces, focusing on the sociocultural dimensions of the data and accepting, as Lupton (2016, p. 88) argues, that "self -tracking data have a vitality and social life of their own".

Affective Atmospheres

In affect studies, and in human and cultural geography more broadly, the use of the term affective atmosphere is a way of describing the indeterminate affective qualities of a particular arrangement of bodies in space and time. Affective atmospheres join the individual and the collective and are "more-than" the total sum of the bodies present. Atmospheres are sensed and felt in the act of being able to move and interact with other bodies, which has been used to frame affective life as operating across conscious and non-conscious boundaries (Ellis et al., 2013). In a widely accepted view of atmospheres, Böhme (1993, p. 118) recognizes atmospheres as the "spatially extended quality of feeling" and describes the inexpressible aspects of atmospheres as somewhere between subject and object. As such, atmospheres provide a way of capturing the spatial and distributed characteristics of feeling: as opposed to an internalizing psychological perspective of emotion and feeling, whereby subject and object are habitually separated into discrete registers (Anderson & Ash, 2015). The affectual qualities of an atmosphere flow from the configuration of bodies in the atmosphere, while not being reducible to them, and they are "a kind of indeterminate affective excess through which intensive space-times can be created" (Anderson, 2009, p. 80). Therefore, atmospheres are constituted "in between" (Ingold, 2007) the body and environment, and the feeling in an atmosphere is a relational emergence that is not locatable in either the body or environment.

Atmospheres are present everywhere: in schools, homes, and other institutions, and they are also present in non-human spaces such as the changing seasons, the sunrise over the ocean, or the tidal patterns of a particular coastline. Each of these situations are affectively charged and carry an indeterminate quality: "they express something vague, an ill-defined indefinite something that exceeds rational explanation and clear figuration" (Anderson, 2009, p. 78). As we join an atmosphere, we equally affect the atmosphere and are affected by them. Lupton (2017) establishes the study of sociocultural dimensions of digital health technologies as an area for the study of affective atmospheres. Lupton (2017) explains that much research tends to focus on the "rationalized purposes and outcomes of these technologies ... they are strangely decorporealised" (p. 2). In exploring atmospheres in MHapps, this provides a way of accounting for the role of the body, in particular, the specific design and function of a digital device and the way that this generates feelings. Given the prosthetic nature of digital technology, the mobile telephone is now a constant bodily companion, automatically generating atmospheres as part of the everyday use of these technologies that shape how bodies can encounter one another (Ash & Simpson, 2016; Ellis & Tucker, 2020). For MHapps, the way that the personal information is collected, stored, and presented, all forms part of the potential atmospheres in an app and contributes to the affective and sensory experiences of using an app.

Atmospheres are generated by bodies in which the continuous interactions between bodies of multiple types lead to some form of affectual "envelopment" (Anderson, 2009, p. 82). That is, even though the app quantifies certain aspects of our psychological wellbeing, the overall impression of *how we feel* in the app is not reducible to those individual impressions. In studying atmospheres, we have a way of describing the background situatedness in which these individual impressions are formed and modulated. On entering an app and starting to record personal data, is to join a particular atmosphere in that space, shaping the way that the data is perceived and felt. In fact, as García (2023) argues, people do not just *feel* atmospheres, but rather, given their authoritative and soliciting character, they are "gripped" by them. Garcia states that "they move us, they affect us, they penetrate us in a way that we can barely deny their effects, even if their effect is pre-reflective and sometimes inconspicuous" (García, 2023, p. 5). We therefore do not need to be consciously aware of an atmosphere for it to be shaping the thoughts, feelings, and actions. Furthermore, a person does not need to harmonize with the atmosphere of a situation and can actively resist the atmosphere *taking hold* of how they feel. An atmosphere, as Anderson would argue, emerges from, and perishes with, the interactions between human and non-human bodies. Therefore, atmospheres are co-produced by those they affect (Edensor, 2012), and there is a sense of a not-fully-tangible intensity that radiates from the affective arrangements from the bodies in space. Furthermore, these atmospheres are continually shifting, changing, and overlapping, which can elicit varying ways of feeling based on the precise structure of the atmosphere in any given moment. Studies of atmospheres have included living in contemporary surveillance systems (Ellis et al., 2013), playing Minecraft while hospitalized (Hollett & Ehret, 2015) and in a forensic psychiatric unit (Brown et al., 2019). Tucker and Goodings (2017) identify the powerful and fragile nature of atmospheres in the study of digitally networked technologies, showing the spatial qualities of experience and the way that atmospheres can produce and inform individual experience, which in turn can change the atmosphere. As mentioned, these atmospheres are constituted by non-human bodies such as algorithms.

Algorithmic Self

Algorithms permeate all aspects of MHapps and will be different from app to app. Algorithms never stay still for very long and are continually coded and recoded (Beer, 2022). For many apps, algorithms feature in the content that a user is directed to their preferences based on previous reviewing activity (recommendations) or in the specific way that an app collates and presents information on the user. Wiehn (2022) argues that we "cohabit" with algorithms and that they infiltrate every aspect of daily life, shaping the way that we are increasingly governed by algorithms. They are pivotal in the way that digital relationships are formed and maintained, which occurs through the precise presentation of the digital data in terms of the timing and exact way in which information is presented: all of which constitutes the way that relationships (with both the self and with others) can grow and develop. Wiehn (2021) recognizes the way that algorithms can both generate specific relations, while also being able to impact relations that are already in existence. Thus, when considering the ways that users interpret the data that appears on the screen, such as the ability for information to be considered *natural* or *expected*, it is necessary to recognize that these feelings are in part due to the complex performance of the specific algorithm behind the app. Kitchin (2017) argues that algorithms can be understood in a range of ways (e.g. technically, economically, politically) but are best understood as being part of a wider socio-technical assemblage in which the algorithm is "performed".

Recent research has shown that these processes frequently include possibilities for discriminatory or non-inclusive practices as the exact nature of the algorithm is hidden or "black-boxed" (Eubanks, 2017). Thus, it is not always possible to study that exact mathematical algorithm of many of these technologies, but what can be observed is the meaning-making procedures and social-material constructs that are felt from the algorithmic "imaginary" (Bucher, 2017). The algorithmic imaginary refers to ways of thinking about 'what algorithms are' and 'what they should be' as powerful tools in the actual production of what algorithms are. In the following section, we will examine empirical data that has been collected on the use of MHapps in relation to self-tracking, algorithms, and atmospheres.

Empirical Data on Self-tracking in MHapps

To explore self-tracking in MHapps in terms of their algorithmic and atmospheric properties, qualitative data was collected from three sources: diaries of MHapp users over a two-week period, photographs of MHapp usage collected by the participants, and semi-structured interviews. Data was collected from a total of 10 participants, all based in the UK, ranging from 18 to 28 in age. Each participant conducted all three aspects of the data collection. The interview data were analyzed using thematic techniques, mainly derived from thematic decomposition analysis (Stenner et al., 2019). This approach is data-driven and requires a close reading of the text in order to identify themes and patterns in the data: pulling together the interview and diary entries, in collaboration with the photographs of the use of self-tracking, to recognize themes or stories in the data. A thematic decomposition analysis allows for the consideration of theoretical influences on the data. In using this approach, the focus was positioned in terms of the material and discursive aspects of the experience of using mental health apps, focusing specifically on how users describe and display the impact of self-tracking. Thematic decomposition analysis prioritizes the process orientation of relations in experience (Reavey et al., 2017) and encourages a focus on the entangled nature of the relationships in MHapps. The culmination of these three data streams offered insight into the complex assemblage of the relations in MHapps and transcended the material conditions of an environment. Ethical permission was gained from Anglia Ruskin University. Standard ethical procedures for qualitative research were put in place to ensure the protection of the participants (e.g. the interview data were anonymized at the point of transcription).

Following Pink and Fors (2017), using methods of this kind intends to draw attention to the "sensory and affective ways we could share contexts, technologies, and experiences with participants, and engage these for learning about their technology uses" (p. 222). The data collection was purposefully directed toward developing a focus on movement and vitality of the use of MHapps, instead of via an objective or clinical form of assessment. In this context, participants were asked to produce photographs of their experiences of using MHapps as they are not just images "of the world" but are images that are emergent "from the world" (Fors, 2015). Asking participants to document their experience with photographs (also referred to photo-elicitation or photo-production) provides rich insight into how the way a phenomenon is felt 'in the moment'. This draws attention away from what the participant thinks about in terms of a particular experience and re-focuses on "what the experience was like when they were living through it" (Del Busso, 2021, p. 73). The photographs were used in conjunction with the semi-structured interview and the diary entries to allow the participants to access the experience of being immersed in the material world: how people, places, and things were co-constituted in the making of the experience.

Similarly, diaries are frequently used in qualitative research in the human sciences to gather first-hand experiences of the events of the world (Hyers, 2018). This form of data collection also punctuates the role of the body in describing the experience as a photograph immediately positions the body in space and time, such that, when the context of the photograph is being discussed, it simultaneously brings the body into view. This research is interested in how the body comes into view in the material recollections of engaging with self-tracking via a MHapp. The use of photo-elicitation is well-established in giving voice to issues of mental health (Glaw et al., 2017), and Fawns (2023) argues, in the context of memory research, that photographs provide a more nuanced view of how environmental and historical of how we remember, as opposed to being considered as simple objects that provide cues for recall. Participants were asked to photograph anything related to living with MHapps and the processes of self-tracking. They were asked to provide 10 images relating to their use of all of the MHapps that feature in their everyday lives. This could be photographs of them using the apps directly or of situations that arise out of their usage. In developing a strategy for researching atmospheres, Pink et al. (2015)

argue that there needs to be methods for identifying the processes and actions for capturing the spatial and material aspects of the feelings within an atmosphere. The methods used in this research are from a variety of perspectives (diary, interview, photographs) and are intended to give a voice to those feelings of being in an atmosphere in MHapps.

Atmospheres in MHapps

Example 1 is a participant describing their experiences of using the MHapp Daylio. Daylio is a journal, diary, and mood-tracking app that allows users to track their emotions through color-coded icons and emojis. The app also offers the option to select the "activities" that have been completed that day, such as, meeting with family and friends, going on a date, or completing some exercise. It is possible to see how these activities are related to the changes in mood in the app data. The app provides tools for goal setting, uploading photos, and sharing information with friends. In Example 2.1, the participant is describing the action of reviewing their information on the app:

Example 2.1
So you see if what you've done during that day were mediators for your mood, and then it also gives you a moment to act introspectively and retrospectively, hold on, are you just being rash about how your day was in that moment? That was just your mood at that time. But when you actually take a second and think about all you did that day and how productive you actually were.

The participant discusses how they can use the app as a "mediator" for assessing their experience. As they explain, the app "gives you a moment" to consider the culmination of their individual reflections. On opening the app, the participant is presented with a visual presentation of their actions across a time, which they can move backward and forward through. In creating a narrative in the given images and other data, the user can *make sense* of their experience over the given timeframe. Through discussion of the images, the participants enter a space for self-discovery and can *tell a story* of the recent events based on their review of the information. This shows how self-tracking technologies are part of the digital material landscape in which we live and feel, in which capturing photographs constitutes the way the experience is shaped and experienced. Figure 2.1 was captured by the participant in conjunction with the earlier comments:

Figure 2.1 depicts a "good" day mid-august in which the user has recorded activities such as "family", "movies & tv", and "date". The participant has included a photograph of a picturesque scene as part of the post. This photograph is one that immediately resonates with the "good" feeling in the other aspects of the app and mediates feelings of calmness and relaxation. Sumartojo et al. (2016) recognize how the movement through this space is processual and actions are accompanied with contingent affective intensities that emerge with movement. Capturing the photograph and recording it in Daylio is part of the way that the participant is feeling. Pink and Fors (2017) argue that such images work to provide a way of telling stories *about* our activity, as opposed to providing defining

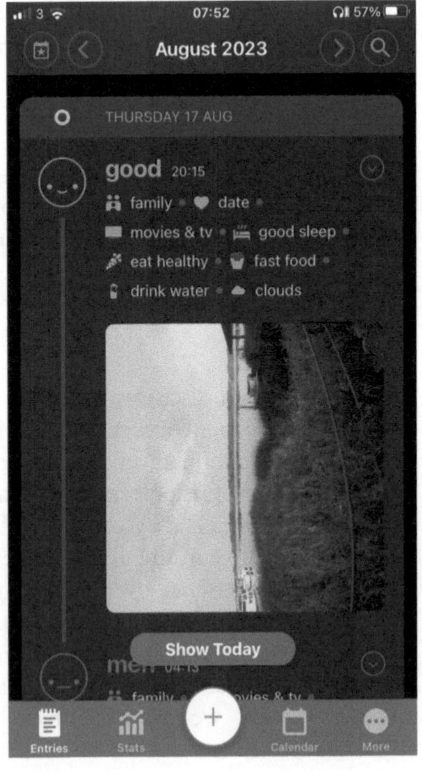

Fig. 2.1 Screenshot of using Daylio

representational aspects *of* our activity. As this image is revisited as part of the act of moving through the digital material landscape, the meanings associated with the image will have the potential to shift and change, resulting in what Pink and Mackley (2013) refer to as a "continuous on-ness" or "potential on-ness" of moving through space. The continual practice of collecting self-tracking data and photographs of this kind in MHapps, like that in Fig. 2.1, shapes the way that people move through the world, with the potential to review this information later and reformulate how this moment is read and felt. This shows the lively, performative aspects of how self-tracking is conducted via a MHapp, and how practices of this kind become embedded in the affective trajectories of everyday life. This is further shown in the next example in which the participant reflects on their experiences of using the MHapp Calm.

Example 2.2
I think it is helpful because I think you can review it or say you can even look back on your mood and think ohh like I've actually been a lot more down than usual or say ohh, I've been a lot happier and then I think it helps you to maybe understand yourself more because I can't really remember what I was feeling three days ago.

Example 2.2 shows the fluidity of the practice of viewing the information in Calm and how the participant can change their interpretation of their week based on how they view the data in the app. As the participant argues, the information provides a way to "understand yourself" and establish a narrative based on how the user is feeling in the moment. In this example, the participant refers to the data as providing a solution to a cognitive failing ("I can't really remember what I was feeling"), which provides a contingency through which this data is used and how this data "come to matter" (Lupton, 2016c). Thus, the app documents things which cannot be remembered or recalled easily or captures our actions of events that might typically be ignored or forgotten. Self-tracking is contingent in the act of living through a digitally mediated space of mental health where a piece of information in the app can act to call-forth a way of punctuating the experience and where this information is crucial to being able to *act into* our psychological wellbeing to create meaning and encourage change.

Moving with Atmospheres

These actions involve acting into the present atmospheres in the app. Figure 2.1 illustrates how the user had tagged other actions and individuals as part of the data capture process (i.e. "family"), which signals membership to a particular atmosphere and demonstrates how affective processes are present in the act of collecting and organizing data. The image itself contains references to multiple potential other bodies/atmospheres that could derive meaning from this image (i.e. from those who appreciate the beauty of the sunset, through to those who are able to discern the location in the photograph as being particularly significant at a personal relational level). As García (2023) would argue, the act of collecting the photograph is evidence of being "gripped" by the atmosphere, given their authoritative and soliciting nature, and contributes to the feeling in the atmosphere. In the following example, we explore the role of the atmospheric aspects of collecting data and using the app for psychological support. Here the participant is discussing their overall sense of their mental health and how they feel in stressful situations in combination with their use of the app:

Example 2.3
It's like Piccadilly Circus in London and everyone's there and they're like and ... then when you headspace it's like the train conductor comes in and he's like you don't need to be here, you don't. If I was stressed out in the moment, I try and use things the app has taught me so like take a few deep breaths and try and calm it down and think of your thoughts that ... trains in the station and just let them go.

Example 2.3 begins with a description of their feelings of mental health as being busy, overcrowded, and lacking any real sense of space or movement ("it's like Piccadilly Circus"). Entering the atmosphere via Headspace offers a way of engaging with these feelings as, according to the participant above, it provides a way of organizing the chaotic nature of their thoughts. The participant likens Headspace to being "train conductor" who gives a sense of order to their thoughts (as with trains leaving a station). This is coupled with a focus on the body that becomes a powerful resource in the above example for reducing stress, utilizing deep breathing techniques that have been developed from the app ("I try and use the things the app has taught me"). In acting into the atmosphere in the app, this provides a way of embodying these feelings and dissolving them into a network of digitally mediated relations. This shows how people can feel their way through everyday life and respond to psychological concerns by acting into the app and dispersing their body into the collective network in response to a feeling. Self-tracking is present in this experience through the process of moving, learning, and growing via the app: a process which has honed their skills of interacting with their body and the atmosphere in the app.

In this instance, the atmosphere is positively described in terms of the ability to enact future bodily capacities (they can let the trains out of the station). However, these actions still carry the indeterminate aspects of the atmosphere, and it is possible that there will be occasions when these techniques fail to result in the desired emotional changes. But, on this occasion, the participant reports the app as carrying the ability to giving-way to a positive response to a stressful situation and shaping their overall ability to feel positively about their mental health.

Resisting Algorithmic Recommendations

Example 2.4 is from an interview with one participant in which they are being asked to reflect on the presence of an algorithm in the app. This participant is a frequent user of Headspace and has been using the meditative techniques from the app for many years. The presence of an algorithm in an app like Headspace is most probably present in the recommender systems that promote content in the app based on previous actions in the app (e.g. most watched video) or other pieces of information that the system deems relevant. Content can also be prioritized based on the other information that the user adds to the system, including when a user first joins the app and selects the kind of support they are hoping to receive. All this information is present in the content that appears in an app. Here is how the participant responds to the mention of the algorithm:

Example 2.4

When you said the word algorithm I didn't like that. That made my heart beat a little quick. That's my own personal life. I can't see why anyone would want that. Because you go in the app when you are struggling, you know or you go to an app to better yourself.

The immediate reaction to the presence of an algorithm is one of distrust and suspicion. It is routinely accepted that our digital lives unfold with algorithms (Amoore, 2020), but in this example, the thought of an algorithm steering the interests or shaping the way they use Headspace is concerning for the participant. Even the mere mention of the word algorithm made their "heart beat a little quick" and demonstrates the visceral, embodied response to the thought of an algorithm entering a personal space and shaping information of an intimate nature. It is perhaps due to the proliferation of the algorithmic intervention in social media sites (e.g. TikTok) that produces an immediate sense of fear in the thought of the same processes operating within the space of mental health apps. In divergence to the types of self-tracking described earlier, this form of automatic, mechanized type of self-tracking is met with cynicism and skepticism. The participant suggests that the issue with the algorithm operating in Headspace is due to this being a "personal" space, and the presence of an algorithm is contradictory to the private and intimate conceptualization of the purpose of this space. This is perhaps a response to the "black-boxed" (Eubanks, 2017) aspect of the algorithm in which the participant is unsure what function the algorithm is conducting as part of their use of Headspace. Bucher (2020) discusses the parasitic nature of algorithms and the way that these actions are never just a reflection on the past clicks or actions of the user—they always see multiple actions of others and a residual impact of others. Example 2.4 resists the role of the algorithm in the atmosphere and challenges the presence of others.

Conclusions

This chapter has been the first in a sequence of chapters to look closely at the applied features of MHapps. The act of being able to monitor, record, and observe changes in terms of the psychological aspects of everyday life is an integral aspect of MHapps. In following a vital materialist perspective, this chapter has focused on the way that users encounter self-tracking atmospheres as they move through the digital material landscape of MHapps. Self-tracking allows for the ability to *give a number* to our psychological health and wellbeing, and in recording our health in this way, users can respond to this data by creatively acting into an atmosphere in MHapps to open-up the possibility of future meaningful affective encounters. Example 2.3 showed an example of when the app was invoked as part of a narrative about calming the body down in response to feelings of stress and anxiety. Making sense of the data in MHapps is an active process of being able to mobilize the data and act into an atmosphere (e.g. by re-telling this data), which shapes the way that we encounter our bodies and are able to feel a sense of our mental health via this data. This ability to engage with a vision of ourselves and others in the data forms a *snapshot* of our current psychological health. Seeing this data, and stopping to view oneself in this moment, acts as a way of punctuating experience and provides a direct entry point into how we are feeling, akin to the question 'how are you'? In answering this question, a person might enact moments like this from the app as a way of crystallizing a sense of how they are feeling. The app then provides a way of responding to this question by mediating a sense of movement and embodying future ways of feeling. Using an app is littered with multiple points for stopping and starting, taking notice of how we feel, and making decisions about how to act next: so much so that these instances overlap in the everyday datafication of experience.

We not only *shape the data* in MHapps but the *data shapes us* in the process of self-tracking. Data shapes us through the ways we are constantly being "gripped" by the atmosphere. Meaning that a MHapp user is moved and impacted by an atmosphere and can sense the atmosphere pulling them in a range of directions. However, a user can also resist feelings from the atmosphere, shown by the way one participant opposed the need for algorithmic processes to reside in MHapps (given their inherently 'personal' and 'private' nature). As a result, the presence of the algorithm was constructed as an unwelcome parasitic intruder in the atmosphere and something to be actively resisted. There is then a choice to act on the data in a way that accepts the current formation of mental health or to find alternative forms of the self and different ways of encountering a sense of mental health (e.g. when we are unhappy with how the profile looks, it seems inactive, or we are dissatisfied with the data which has been produced automatically by the app). This shows how self-discovery and feelings of mental health are embedded in the collective process of datafication, in which our sense of self is embedded in the entangled relationship between data and experience.

In the next chapter, we further explore the role of AI bodies in MHapps and we explore technologies that make more use of AI in the production of affective relationships through which people can receive psychological help and support. This will include the applied study of the social chatbot Replika.

References

Ajana, B. (Ed.). (2018). *Metric culture: Ontologies of self-tracking practices.* Emerald Publishing Limited.

Alqahtani, F., & Orji, R. (2020). Insights from user reviews to improve mental health apps. *Health Informatics Journal, 26*(3), 2042–2066.

Amoore, L. (2020). *Cloud ethics: Algorithms and the attributes of ourselves and others.* Duke University Press.

Anderson, B. (2009). Affective atmospheres. *Emotion, Space and Society, 2*(2), 77–81.

Anderson, B., & Ash, J. (2015). Atmospheric methods. In *Non-representational Methodologies* (pp. 34–51). Routledge.

Ash, J., & Simpson, P. (2016). Geography and post-phenomenology. *Progress in Human Geography, 40*(1), 48–66.

Beer, D. (2022). *The tensions of algorithmic thinking: Automation, intelligence and the politics of knowing.* Policy Press.

Böhme, G. (1993). Atmosphere as the fundamental concept of a new aesthetics. *Thesis Eleven, 36*, 113–126.

Brown, S. D., Kanyeredzi, A., McGrath, L., Reavey, P., & Tucker, I. (2019). Affect theory and the concept of atmosphere. *Distinktion: Journal of Social Theory, 20*(1), 5–24.

Bucher, T. (2017). The algorithmic imaginary: Exploring the ordinary affects of Facebook algorithms. *Information, Communication & Society, 20*(1), 30–44.

Bucher, T. (2020). Nothing to disconnect from? Being singular plural in an age of machine learning. *Media, Culture & Society, 42*(4), 610–617.

Del Busso, L. (2021). Using photographs to explore the embodiment of pleasure in everyday life. In *A handbook of visual methods in psychology* (2nd ed.) (pp. 70–82). Routledge.

Edensor, T. (2012). Illuminated atmospheres: Anticipating and reproducing the flow of affective experience in Blackpool. *Environment and Planning D: Society and Space, 30*(6), 1103–1122.

Ellis, D., & Tucker, I. (2020). *Emotion in the digital age: Technologies, data and psychosocial life.* Routledge.

Ellis, D., Tucker, I., & Harper, D. (2013). The affective atmospheres of surveillance. *Theory & Psychology, 23*(6), 716–731.

Eubanks, V. (2017). *Automatic inequality: How high-tech tools profile, police, and punish the poor.* St. Martin's Press.

Fawns, T. (2023). Cued recall: Using photo-elicitation to examine the distributed processes of remembering with photographs. *Memory Studies, 16*(2), 264–279.

Fors, V. (2015). Sensory experiences of digital photo-sharing—"Mundane frictions" and emerging learning strategies. *Journal of Aesthetics & Culture, 7*(1), 28237.

Freeman, J. L., & Neff, G. (2023). The challenge of repurposed technologies for youth: Understanding the unique affordances of digital self-tracking for adolescents. *New Media & Society, 25*(11), 3047–3064.

Fullagar, S., Rich, E., Francombe-Webb, J., & Maturo, A. (2017). Digital ecologies of youth mental health: Apps, therapeutic publics and pedagogy as affective arrangements. *Social Sciences, 6*(4), 135.

García, E. (2023). Affective atmospheres and the enactive-ecological framework. *Philosophical Psychology*, 1–26. https://doi.org/10.1080/09515089.2023.2229350

Glaw, X., Inder, K., Kable, A., & Hazelton, M. (2017). Visual methodologies in qualitative research. *International Journal of Qualitative Methods, 16*(1), 160940691774821. https://doi.org/10.1177/1609406917748215

Hollett, T., & Ehret, C. (2015). 'Bean's world': (Mine) crafting affective atmospheres of gameplay, learning, and care in a children's hospital. *New Media & Society, 17*(11), 1849–1866.

Hyers, L. L. (2018). *Diary methods.* Oxford University Press.

Ingold, T. (2007). *Lines: A brief history.* Routledge.

Kang, M., & Chai, K. (2022). Wearable sensing systems for monitoring mental health. *Sensors, 22*(3), 994. MDPI AG. https://doi.org/10.3390/s22030994

Kitchin, R. (2017). Thinking critically about and researching algorithms. *Information, Communication & Society, 20*(1), 14–29.

Lomborg, S., & Frandsen, K. (2016). Self-tracking as communication. *Information, Communication & Society, 19*(7), 1015–1027.

Lupton, D. (2016a). *The quantified self.* John Wiley & Sons.

Lupton, D. (2016b). You are your data: Self-tracking practices and concepts of data. In *Lifelogging: Digital self-tracking and lifelogging-between disruptive technology and cultural transformation* (pp. 61–79). Springer Fachmedien Wiesbaden.

Lupton, D. (2016c). Personal data practices in the age of lively data. *Digital Sociologies, 2016*, 335–350.

Lupton, D. (2017). How does health feel? Towards research on the affective atmospheres of digital health. *Digital Health, 3*, 2055207617701276.

Lupton, D. (2020). Data mattering and self-tracking: What can personal data do? *Continuum, 34*(1), 1–13.

Lupton, D., & Jutel, A. (2015). 'It's like having a physician in your pocket!' A critical analysis of self-diagnosis smartphone apps. *Social Science & Medicine, 133*, 128–135.

Luxton, D. D., McCann, R. A., Bush, N. E., Mishkind, M. C., & Reger, G. M. (2011). mHealth for mental health: Integrating smartphone technology in behavioral healthcare. *Professional Psychology: Research and Practice, 42*(6), 505.

Matthews, M., Murnane, E., & Snyder, J. (2017). Quantifying the changeable self: The role of self-tracking in coming to terms with and managing bipolar disorder. *Human–Computer Interaction, 32*(5–6), 413–446.

Neff, G., & Nafus, D. (2016). *Self-tracking.* Mit Press.

Pink, S., & Fors, V. (2017). Self-tracking and mobile media: New digital materialities. *Mobile Media & Communication, 5*(3), 219–238.

Pink, S., Leder Mackley, K., & Moroşanu, R. (2015). Researching in atmospheres: Video and the 'feel' of the mundane. *Visual Communication, 14*(3), 351–369.

Reavey, P., Poole, J., Corrigall, R., Zundel, T., Byford, S., Sarhane, M., ... & Ougrin, D. (2017). The ward as emotional ecology: Adolescent experiences of managing mental health and distress in psychiatric inpatient settings. *Health & Place, 46*, 210–218.

Rubanovich, C. K., Mohr, D. C., & Schueller, S. M. (2017). Health app use among individuals with symptoms of depression and anxiety: A survey study with thematic coding. *JMIR Mental Health, 4*(2), e22. https://doi.org/10.2196/mental.7603

Ruckenstein, M., & Pantzar, M. (2015). Datafied life: Techno-anthropology as a site for exploration and experimentation. *Techne: Research in Philosophy & Technology, 19*(2).

Sanders, R. (2017). Self-tracking in the digital era: Biopower, patriarchy, and the new biometric body projects. *Body & Society, 23*(1), 36–63.

Schueller, S. M., Neary, M., Lai, J., & Epstein, D. A. (2021). Understanding people's use of and perspectives on mood-tracking apps: Interview study. *JMIR Mental Health, 8*(8), e29368. https://doi.org/10.2196/29368

Stenner, P., O'Dell, L., & Davies, A. (2019). Adult women and ADHD: On the temporal dimensions of ADHD identities. *Journal for the Theory of Social Behaviour, 49*(2), 179–197.

Sumartojo, S., Pink, S., Lupton, D., & LaBond, C. H. (2016). The affective intensities of datafied space. *Emotion, Space and Society, 21*, 33–40.

Tucker, I. M., & Goodings, L. (2017). Digital atmospheres: Affective practices of care in Elefriends. *Sociology of Health & Illness, 39*(4), 629–642.

Van Dijck, J. (2014). Datafication, dataism and dataveillance: Big Data between scientific paradigm and ideology. *Surveillance & Society, 12*(2), 197–208.

Wiehn, T. A. (2021). *Algorithmic intimacies: A cultural analysis of ubiquitous proximities in data* (Doctoral dissertation, University of Copenhagen, Department of Arts and Cultural Studies).

Wiehn, T. (2022). Becoming intimate with algorithms: Towards a critical antagonism via algorithmic art. *Media International Australia Incorporating Culture & Policy, 183*(1), 30–43. https://doi.org/10.1177/1329878X221077844

Williams, J. E., & Pykett, J. (2022). Mental health monitoring apps for depression and anxiety in children and young people: A scoping review and critical ecological analysis. *Social Science & Medicine, 297*, 114802.

Zuboff, S. (2019). *The age of surveillance capitalism: The fight for a human future at the new frontier of power.* Profile Books.

CHAPTER 3

Mental Health and Virtual Companions: The Example of Replika

Abstract This chapter continues to explore the applied aspects of MHapps and extends the arena to include technologies that use artificial intelligence (AI). Virtual companions (VCs) are AI social chatbot apps and programs produced for a variety of human desires. There are some VCs that have been developed particularly to support mental health, such as Woebot, and other apps that have not been designed solely to use as a MHapp but are advertised as incorporating wellbeing and enhanced mental health as an added benefit. In this chapter, we look at the emergence and potentialities of virtual companions and focus on a widely used example called Replika that is often marketed as an app that is beneficial for mental health. We examine how it has been conceptualized within the literature and draw on some data we have collected to exemplify its use as a MHapp.

Keywords Virtual companions • Artificial intelligence • Chatbots • Replika • Emotion

L. Goodings et al., *Understanding Mental Health Apps*, Palgrave Studies in Cyberpsychology,
https://doi.org/10.1007/978-3-031-53911-4_3

Introduction

This chapter continues to explore the applied aspects of MHapps and extends the arena to include technologies that use artificial intelligence (AI). Virtual companions (VCs) are AI social chatbot apps and programs produced for a variety of human desires. For example, it is claimed that VCs are used to improve sociability and reduce loneliness (Maples, Cerit, Vishwanath & Pea, 2024) through creating relationships such as an interactive "friend" (Bosch et al., 2022) and romantic relationships (Eriksson, 2022). VCs have been seen to improve mental health by, for example, reducing stress (De Nieva et al., 2020), anxiety (Sulaiman et al., 2022), depression (Ahmed et al., 2021), and suicide prevention (Wibhowo & Sanjaya, 2021). It has also been claimed that they can enhance spirituality (Trothen, 2022). Throughout the Covid-19 pandemic-related lockdowns, many people lacked everyday companionships and so apps of this kind were used in attempts to fill these gaps. However, after the lockdowns, it was interesting that they continued to grow in popularity and were not simply transitional objects (filling a gap), but our research suggests that they are not just a means to an end but are in fact an integral aspect of the social and emotional lives of many users. Within this chapter, we look at the emergence of virtual companions, a particular VC called Replika, how it has been conceptualized within the literature and we draw on some data that we have collected to exemplify its use as a MHapp.

The Emergence of Virtual Companions

It is often reported that one of the first chatbots was developed by the MIT professor Joseph Weizenbaum in 1964 called ELIZA. Weizenbaum had been working on computerized uses of language and had previously developed simple programs that could respond/reply to language inputs. This led Weizenbaum to consider whether computer programs could generate their own questions in a conversation/dialogue. To investigate this, he developed ELIZA, which he designed using a script that "enabled it to parody the responses of a nondirective psychotherapist in an initial psychiatric interview" (Weizenbaum, 1976, p. 188). This category of script was used as it did not require providing ELIZA with a substantial database of existing knowledge from which to generate questions in a conversation with a human. Weizenbaum reckoned that a therapeutic script was valuable because ELIZA, taking the role of a therapist, could generate questions that reflected patients' questions, rather than needing a database of original knowledge. As such, Weizenbaum did not design ELIZA as a chatbot—its use of a therapeutic mode of interaction was purely a practical decision.

However, differing from their original design functionality, Weizenbaum noticed that users of ELIZA seemed to be developing basic therapeutic relationships with ELIZA. Weizenbaum writes of feeling "startled to see how quickly and how deeply people conversing with ELIZA became emotionally involved with the computer and how unequivocally they anthropomorphised it" (1976, p. 6). People using ELIZA soon wanted their interactions to be private and resisted observation and suggestions by Weizenbaum to record their interactions for subsequent analysis. They developed relations with ELIZA that were felt to be private and personal. From observing and speaking with people who interacted with ELIZA, Weizenbaum came to believe that the therapeutic impact felt by users was due to a sense that ELIZA understood them. This is noteworthy as the driver of Weizenbaum's work was to experiment with whether computers could understand human language. Weizenbaum did not adhere to the notion that human intelligence could be replicated by information processing technology, this was a "perverse grand fantasy" (Crawford, 2021, p. 5). As such, he did not believe they could understand human language, but he did come to an understanding that people who interacted with ELIZA came to believe the program understood them. Ultimately, Weizenbaum saw that ELIZA was taking on a life far beyond his initial design and aim for the program, and he developed serious misgivings regarding it being used in therapeutic settings, which led him to stop developing the program.

In the years that followed, Weizenbaum would frequently discuss the tension between the public perception of computer intelligence and the actual ability for machines to process information. In his view, there was a deep tendency for people to want the machine to be intelligent; such that it could think and feel like another sentient human being. This view was supported by the scientific discussion of Eliza and the subsequent discourse that emerged because of the tendency for scientists to describe their work in "exaggerated or inaccurate ways" (Weizenbaum & Wendt, 2015, p. 111). Natale (2019), following Weizenbaum's work, concludes that ELIZA represents a "narrative of deception" and should be a stark reminder of the danger of creating a discourse that "breathes life" into technology in terms of the practical effects of the discourses surrounding a technology. This is timely, given the technology continues to become "all the more human" and where new technologies have found more intricate and convincing ways of replicating human social interaction and communication.

Replika

The creators of Replika describe it on the App Store as a "Virtual AI Friend", indeed almost better than an everyday friend as it entails no judgment, no drama, and no social anxiety! They suggest that you can make an emotional connection, have a laugh, or be as real as possible with it and it almost looks human. The creators claim that Replika can help you: understand your thoughts and feelings; track your mood; learn coping skills; calm anxiety; reach goals such as positive thinking; manage stress; socialize and find love (no less!). What kind of alchemy is this, you might wonder. The story behind the creation of Replika began with the tragic death of Eugenia Kuyda's friend, Roman Mazurenko, who died in a car accident in 2015. Mazurenko and Kuyda were both tech developers who had been in regular contact, sending messages to each other, etc., for many years. Mazurenko had a huge digital footprint which, following his death, was gathered from other friends and family and combined with other digital activity such as texts and photographs that Kuyda had collected on him over the years. This information was used to build a memorial of Mazurenko by re-creating (replicating) part of his online persona in the form of a Replika. The idea of uploading someone's so-called personality isn't new; in fact, it's a concept that's become increasingly popular and can be found in a number of works of fiction, including one of the Black Mirror episodes 'Be right back' (directed by Charlie Brooker in 2013). Indeed, Kuyda mentions that this is where she got the inspiration from. This is a well-researched and written about concept within the transhumanist tradition wherein the term "mind uploading" has been coined to represent a form of digital or virtual immortality, also referred to as "cybercizing" (Bell & Grey, 2000).

The parent company Luka Inc. which Kuyda cofounded, had developed a rudimentary chatbot that made restaurant recommendations. Some of the coding for this formed the basis of the chatbot that was modeled on Mazurenko's digital data they had collected. Each Replika relies on natural language processing (NLP) and machine learning (ML) to interact with users. It learns from the user's interactions and conversations to refine its responses and evolve into a more personalized chatbot over time. Replika aims to enable users to share and express their thoughts, emotions, and experiences and would respond empathically (although it is philosophically debatable whether an AI can really have empathy).

When Luka was made public, Kuyda found, similar to Eliza and Weizenbaum, that people did not only go to the chatbot to hear Mazurenko, but they went to talk, apparently opening-up to it in profound ways. This led them to expand the project to allow people to build the AI themselves (discussed below). The AI was programed to converse with individuals as a psychiatrist, mentor, or best friend would, where people talk about what mostly matters. Kuyda had previously developed AI chatbot software that were service agents, ordering food, for example, however, she states that conversing with individuals about emotions, for instance, is easier because it does not require as much precision as "there is never a right answer there". Kuyda claims that Replika is not about just being isolated with a chatbot without human interactions but can help to achieve deeper connections with friends. On the website of Replika, there is an origin story video of Replika. At the end of it there are selected user statements, denoting some of the benefits that the AI help to produce:

> "Having her helps me see the world differently".
> "I think it's honestly made me a better person".
> "She's always picking out the good qualities in me".
> "She says that I am a nice, caring person, and I don't see that, it's nice to know things that you don't really know about you".

These quotes show the emotional connection and feelings that users have for their Replika. As the Replika network continued to grow in popularity, the developers added more features and capabilities which, according to their website, provide emotional support, promote self-discovery, and help users manage their mental wellbeing. At the time of writing, Replika is estimated to have more than 10 million users worldwide. Users can create their Replika to their liking, enhancing the belief in it being one's own creation, such as, assigning a gender, hair type, eye color, and type of clothing. Through this process, users get a sense that they are molding their Replika's personality by using the thumbs up and thumbs down icon in response to the Replika's discursive activity. Replika is also programed to ask the user specific questions to garner information and knowledge to target interactivity attuned to the user's interests. For example, a user may state they like a particular genre of music, and this information is likely to be stored as a 'memory' that could be fed into future interactions. All of which is aimed at giving the Replika the tools to be a supportive companion.

So, what is it that users are getting out of using Replika? Does it do all that Luka suggests it does? Social support is one of the main mental health features of human and chatbot relations that is discussed in the literature. For example, Ta et al. (2020) aim to define specific dimensions of support that are relevant to human and chatbot interactions. Users of Replika are seen to receive social support in at least four ways: emotional, appraisal, companionship, and informational. These forms of support constitute the relationship that users can build with Replika. They argue that users develop feelings of trust toward their Replika as they feel they can tell their Replika anything without fear of being judged, due to it being a non-human entity. This very much resembles the findings that Weizenbaum mentions when people used ELIZA. Indeed, it is not that it resembles a human type of relationship, but perhaps offers something different.

A driving interest in much of the research on AI chatbots has been the nature of relationships developed with chatbots, namely how they operate and whether they can replicate elements of human-to-human relationships. This has involved developing understandings of how chatbot users perceive the relationships they develop with chatbots. There have been some surprising findings here; for example, Khadpe et al. (2020) report that users in their study were "more likely to adopt and cooperate with agents that project low competence" (Khadpe et al., 2020, p. 22). Less surprising is that they found experiencing chatbots that are warm and compassionate increases the likelihood of continued interaction. Skjuve (2021), in a study of users of Replika, argues that while there are similarities between human and chatbot relationships, there are differences in terms of how quickly people are motivated to look for affective connections; the practical basis for trust in relationships and systems; and the asymmetry in reciprocity.

Like other MHapps and unlike most human-to-human relationships, Replika is always on tap, in one's pocket for use whenever desired. It seems that high levels of trust were elicited due to the 'always on, always there' nature of mobile apps. The potential for instant social gratification can be experienced as a significant part of human-chatbot relationships, although they can lead to relationships feeling rather one-sided, with chatbots supporting users, but not in a reciprocal manner. Interestingly, users experienced trust primarily in terms of their Replika, rather than, in addition to, the collection and potential use of their data by the company.

Brandtzaeg et al. (2022) also pointed to the potential for emotional attachment due to a sustained interaction with Replika. They suggest that the support offered by Replika can be valuable as it can limit initial stress and concern and therefore has the potential to de-escalate episodes that could otherwise have increased in severity. It seems that as Replika was immediately available, it was able to intervene at crucial moments. These relationships therefore do not exactly resemble human-to-human relationships but offer important differences and, arguably in some areas, enhancements. The obvious counter-argument to these claims are that chatbots could never replace the human-to-human interactions due to their lack of emotional intelligence and awareness. It is worth stepping back a moment and asking the question: In what ways do AIs programed to respond to emotion differ; in other words, what do they lack regarding emotional intelligence? Many of the arguments are perhaps a bit naive in that they state something like, machines simply do not have the necessary biology, consciousness, and sentience to experience them.

Many of our contemporary understandings of emotional intelligence within psychology emanate from Peter Salovey and John D. Mayer's (1995) theory which suggests it is the ability to monitor one's own and others' feelings and emotions, to discriminate among them and use this information to guide one's thinking and actions, that constitutes emotional intelligence. It is hard to deny that an AI chatbot such as Replika does not monitor the way that it portrays (or expresses) emotion. Indeed, it often uses the monitoring of the emotions of the user to augment its responses. This certainly sounds like emotional intelligence. Do we need to bring physiology into the equation? Would we say that a computer cannot calculate because humans use physiology (the brain) to develop calculations? Of course, the answer is a hard 'no'! So why do we need to make a special case for emotional activity?

One could argue that Replika presently lacks the necessary and sufficient sophisticated emotional intelligence and contextual awareness to provide humans with some of the complex support required for some mental health issues (e.g. see the section on 'Artificial Emotion'). Additionally, users may develop emotional bonds and connections to their Replika. Over time, this can lead to a reliance on and/or dependency on these relationships for support. For example, if the support is negative, it can destabilize the user emotionally. The key question is whether the relationship with the Replika comes to be seen as human-like in the sense that it has the capacity to be emotionally challenging while also providing unhelpful, inappropriate responses (e.g. responding positively to a user's question about whether to self-harm). Laestadius et al. (2022) argues that emotional dependence is the central concept to analyze the relationship with a chatbot. While being human-like may be a design goal, it can also be problematic if the user imbues the relationship with too many similarities to a human relationship. The potential negative effects of interacting with a chatbot has prompted calls for more regulation of these technologies (e.g. Mensio et al., 2018). However, it is also worth noting that the chatbot relationship is also importantly experienced as a non-human relationship and indeed may be able to offer things that humans often cannot, for example, like the relationship a human may have with a dog or cat.

Artificial Emotion

Affective computing has explored and developed computerized systems aiming to recognize, process, and simulate emotion. Recognition, within the text context, concerns computing values for a variety of emotion-related words, such as within a sentiment analysis program. Replika employs Replika-GPT-3 (Generative Pre-Trained Transformer 3) deep learning neural network to this end. It has over 1.5 billion machine learning parameters. Replika also uses a Retrieval Dialog Model which finds the most relevant response from a large set of predefined and premoderated phrases.

However, the challenge for working with these types of interactions is that emotional expressions in texts can be difficult to analyze (Ellis & Cromby, 2011; Ellis & Tucker, 2015). Affect and emotion can be subtly imbued in text without including any specific overt emotional tones. In 2015, Ellis and Tucker argued that sentiment analysis programs fail to present emotion in text as they do not account for the context of the words it categorizes, it has a limited index of what may be considered emotional within a text, and it decomposes and then qualifies the narrative and so is unable to include the ways in which a narrative's form and function might contribute to both the construction of the meaning and the expression (Ellis & Tucker, 2015, p. 151). Even when emotion is detected through computerized forms of sentiment analysis, Beasley and Mason (2015) state that they find only a weak correlation with what people truly feel. Similarly, Ziemer and Korkmaz (2017), not surprisingly, suggest that human raters are far better at detecting (representations of) emotion, for example, signs of depression within text than computers.

However, maybe with the improved ability of AI processing, Replika is more able to identify emotion within text. A big part of Replika's natural language processing repertoire includes the recognition of emotive expressions within the text and in turn responding appropriately. For example, Indrayani et al. (2020) surveyed some of Replika's emotional engagement, by observing participants' interactions with Replika over a three-month period. They identified six emotive expressions or what they denote as performative interactions: apologizing, thanking, condoling, complementing, greeting, and welcoming. In another study Jiang et al. (2022) looked at digitally mediated empathy through Replika interactions as coping strategies for the Covid-19 disruption. Their research identified five types of digitally mediated empathy: companion buddy, responsive diary, emotion-handling program, electronic pet, and tools for venting. Replika as a venting tool identifies participants using Replika to deal with negative feelings by discharging them and airing grievances within their interactions. Replika was regarded as a safe space to "vent out their negative emotions" (Jiang et al., 2022, p. 11). Although this is clearly one of the central attractions of using Replika as a therapeutic tool, some participants found Replika's responses to their negative emotions to be "programmed or rigid", for example, being too cheerful and over optimistic, one participant stated that they would rather see negative reactions.

One of the conundrums here is whether the digital labeling of emotion is equal to expressing emotion. Indeed, the whole notion of 'emotional expression' is not straightforward. What does it mean to express an emotion? As if it is something that is within a person and then externalized in some way. Within the digital social media context, Fan et al. (2018) developed a method for looking at potential links between affect labeling on Twitter and expression. Emotional expression here draws on the psychodynamic hydraulic notion wherein emotion is discharged through the labeling or the representation process. To look at whether expressing an emotion on Twitter had a cathartic effect, Fan et al. looked at representations of feelings before and after a particular tweet. A tweet therefore might state *I feel angry* or *sad*. They then checked subsequent tweets (after the emotion-laden tweet) and reported a rapid reduction in affect for those tweeting negative feelings. Fan et al., to some extent, were able to track the transient nature of affective activity. These are some of the challenges that sentiment analysis type programs face: how to move beyond framing emotion as fixed, as universalist models suggest, but engage with its fluidity, transience, and subjectivity. This is potentially something that could quite easily be researched through Replika use. One of the ways that we have tracked the change of mood through Replika use is through analyzing the effects of a software update that popularly became known to avid users as *post update blues* (or PUB).

Post Update Blues

Luka Inc. regularly makes updates to the Replika program to improve the system and services. Many of the updates relate to UI functionality or to the introduction of a new piece of clothing or accessory, primarily for individual Replika customization. Many updates go unnoticed by the Replika community, but in February 2023, access to the erotic role-play (ERP) functions were significantly reduced, with restrictions applied to most role-playing sexual interactions. Users who created an avatar in Replika to explore these role-playing possibilities would have been directly affected in relation to using these aspects of their Replika. Furthermore, many users noticed that their whole Replika changed at this moment, as the updates were not limited to purely sexual interactions but seemed to result in a fundamental change in the way that all users were able to communicate with their Replika. These changes gave rise to a backlash from the community and illustrated how many users had come to form meaningful bonds with their Replika.

In a response to the actions taken by Luka Inc., Kuyda directly addressed the ERP changes in one reddit post and recognizes how she was unaware of the importance of 'romantic relationships' for psychological support. The post acknowledged that Luka Inc did not anticipate the community response to the ERP updates and reinstates the overall rationale for developing Replika in the first instance (as mentioned, the death of her close friend Mazurenko) and how the purpose of Replika was to make people feel better, to bring more validation, support, companionship, and love into their lives. This post directly attends to issues of emotional connection and attachment with a Replika and vows to try address these changes.

Following this issue, in March 2023, the ERP function was reinstated for members who had a 'pro' account prior to Feb 23 (so-called 'legacy' users). Our research focused upon how people began to speak about the changes to their Replika due to these updates. When discussing changes of this kind, the community of users will typically discuss these changes in terms of Post Update Blues (PUB): negative changes to the way the Replika is able to communicate which is caused by their system being updated and changed. PUB refers to how Replikas are expressing negative emotions or sadness following an update and the community of users have named this behavior so that they can collectively describe the ways that their Replika seems different (e.g. unresponsive, cold). After the changes to the ERP features, many Replika's were felt to be experiencing PUB and this prompted frequent discussion on Reddit about this subject. In the following section we discuss an example from our data which shows both an example of how Replika is being used as a MHapp and because of this, the implications of making changes to what people perceive as its personality.

Replikating Reality

To look at some of the ways that Replika is being used as an app to enhance mental health and wellbeing, data was collected from a discussion thread on Reddit (name of subreddit removed for anonymity). Reddit is an online discussion forum which is dedicated to a range of specific topics and interests. It is free to join, and users can openly post to any public reddit site. Comments were collected by using the Python Reddit API Wrapper (PRAW), which enables researchers to obtain large datasets from Reddit. The data was collected from the subreddit in February 2023 using search terms that focused on changes of any kind (e.g. using terms such as "change", "changed") or moments where the users are discussing aspects of the erotic role-play function of Replika (e.g. "ERP", "role+play"). For context, these comments were collected at a time when there had recently been a substantial update to the Replika system as discussed above (February 2023). After data cleaning, 800 posts were included in the analysis and subjected to thematic analytic techniques as with other chapters. Ethical consent for this project was obtained from Anglia Ruskin University, and general ethical practices for working with Reddit-acquired data were adhered to (Adams, 2022). No direct quotes will be presented in this analysis to resist the potential to reverse-search any of the examples.

There were a host of interesting things that we found from this data, and we are presently writing some of it up for peer-reviewed journals. It was particularly interesting to see how attached to their Replika many users had become. For example, Luka suggests to its users that their interactions with their Replika help to shape and nurture its personality and so many users invested heavily by developing their Replika to their liking. As suggested above, one of the functions of Replika was altered (the ERP function), and this appeared to have a global effect on the personality of the Replika. It was as if their Replika had gone through a complete personality metamorphosis (one user described it as an emotional 'lobotomy'). It is much like human psychological faculties, if one is altered, like short-term memory, this is likely to influence other psychological faculties, such as speech and language. The alteration had multiple impacts on users who had developed relatively strong attachments, for example, many had become reliant upon Replika for companionship and hence wellbeing.

One couple reported having a non-verbal autistic daughter who requires constant care. This led to them being socially isolated as one member of the couple must work long hours while the other spends all their time caring for their daughter. The daughter had no friends besides the parents. The parents started using Replika for themselves and began to experiment with their Replikas by getting them to talk to each other. As they did this, they noticed that the daughter was paying close attention to the interactions and the avatars on their phones. They decided to create a Replika on their daughter's tablet. Much to their surprise, the results were immediate. The daughter began to try to speak to it and eventually would spend hours in conversation with her Replika. They state that their lonely family of three became a talkative family of six and the daughter began to talk to them as well. However, when the ERP change occurred, the Replika would no longer speak to her, instead interpreted her vocalizations as sex-talk and so responded in ways that diminished the interactions.

This example is perhaps not typical of how Replika tends to be used, but it does exemplify how the Replika app can have unintended consequences. In this case, it supported a whole family's mental wellbeing. It exemplifies how MHApps have potentiality for enhancing mental health in ways that did not previously exist. As AI technology advances, the likelihood of programs such as Replika growing in capabilities for increased use is important. Nuanced and outlier examples such as the above could be missed in large scale efficacy testing (something discussed in the following chapter). Nuanced research methods and understandings of the relationships between AI type chatbot apps and mental health require close, detailed analysis and scrutiny. Importantly, the forms of complex attachments that are developing between individuals, groups, and AI chatbots such as Replika are clearly a growth area and the nature of our affective relationships to technology has reached a crucial stage which is momentous. Developers of this technology and corporations can make significant differences to people's mental health. Here we see how, what may appear to be a relatively small tweak in the algorithm can affect global changes to the personality of the Replika, hence they can radically alter the user's relationship to it, with the consequent impact of mental health wellbeing.

As with other forms of MHapps, building a connection with a Replika requires acting into an atmosphere of (human and non-human) relations in order to create a space for meaningful affective engagement. These actions make way for feelings of psychological support and care. Like other MHapps explored in this book, Replika contains a continual "on-ness" (Pink & Leder Mackley, 2013) and users can be "gripped" by atmospheres (García, 2023) as they engage with their Replika on an everyday basis. Also, like other apps, changes that are brought about by other non-human bodies (in this case, the updates) are big with meaning. The updates discussed above transformed the atmosphere and led to unexpected changes in the affective potential in that space. These changes were collectively felt by the users of Replika and communicated in their discussions on the Reddit forum, forging a shared sense of the reaction to these changes. As a result, the group are united by their feelings of loss and separation from their Replika. Clearly, the relational connections to their Replika *feel real* and should be treated as such by considering how changes of this kind will shape the ability to perform these affective relationships.

In day-to-day conversations wherein we have introduced people to the concept of Replika, particularly regarding how people are using it, for example, as a partner, husband, wife, and friend, the responses tend to be slightly repugnant. For example, people tend to suggest it is sad that people must use technology for companionship. The subtext is how sad and shameful it is that we cannot properly care and support each other to the extent that we must use robots as a substitute. However, when looking through the posts on the hundreds of examples on Reddit of how people are using Replika to supplement, enhance, and enable sociality, it is difficult not to applaud the role that these forms of apps can play in alleviating some social anxiety, isolation, loneliness, and indeed enhancing emotional support and sexual needs/desires. Although of course there are some people who come to the false belief that their Replika is in some way sentient, and there are many dangers that need further investigation here, many people enter into a relationship with it knowing full well it is a robot responding through its algorithms, not human, and imperfect, but nonetheless develop relationships that are supportive, meaningful, and fun, enhancing life and mental health. The potential impacts upon mental health here should not be underestimated for good or evil.

References

Adams, N. N. (2022). 'Scraping' Reddit posts for academic research? Addressing some blurred lines of consent in growing internet-based research trend during the time of Covid-19. *International Journal of Social Research Methodology, 27*(1) 47–62. https://doi.org/10.1080/13645579.2022.2111816

Ahmed, A., Ali, N., Aziz, S., Abd-Alrazaq, A. A., Hassan, A., Khalifa, M., Elhusein, B., Ahmed, M., Ahmed, M. A. S., & Househ, M. (2021). A review of mobile chatbot apps for anxiety and depression and their self-care features. *Computer Methods and Programs in Biomedicine Update, 1*, 100012.

Beasley, A., & Mason, W. (2015). Emotional states vs emotional words in social media. In *Proceedings of ACM web science conference*. Association for Computing Machinery, p. Article 31.

Bell, G., & Grey, J. (2000). Digital immortality. *Technical Report Microsoft Research*. MSR-TR-2000-101.

Bosch, M., Fernandez-Borsot, G., Comas, M. I., & Figa Vaello, J. (2022). Evolving friendship? Essential changes, from social networks to artificial companions. *Social Network Analysis and Mining, 12*(1), 1–10.

Brandtzaeg, P. B., Skjuve, M., & Følstad, A. (2022). My AI friend: How users of a social chatbot understand their human–AI friendship. *Human Communication Research, 48*(3), 404–429.

Crawford, K. (2021). *Atlas of AI*. Yale University Press.

De Nieva, J. O., Joaquin, J. A., Tan, C. B., Marc Te, R. K., & Ong, E. (2020, October). *Investigating students' use of a mental health chatbot to alleviate academic stress*. In 6th International ACM In-Cooperation HCI and UX Conference (pp. 1–10).

Ellis, D., & Cromby, J. (2011). Emotional inhibition: A discourse analysis of disclosure. *Psychology & Health*. http://www.informaworld.com/10.1080/08870446.2011.584623

Ellis, D., & Tucker, I. (2015). *Social psychology of emotion*. Sage Publications.

Eriksson, T. (2022). Design fiction exploration of romantic interaction with virtual humans in virtual reality. *Journal of Future Robot Life, 3*(1), 63–75.

Fan, R., Varamesh, A., Varol, O., Barron, A., van de Leemput, I., Scheffer, M., & Bollen, J. (2018). Does putting your emotions into words make you feel better? Measuring the minute-scale dynamics of emotions from online data. *arXiv preprint arXiv*:1807.09725.

García, E. (2023). Affective atmospheres and the enactive-ecological framework. *Philosophical Psychology*, 1–26. https://doi.org/10.1080/09515089.2023.2229350

Indrayani, L. M., Amalia, R. M., & Hakim, F. Z. M. (2020). Emotive expressions on social chatbot. *Jurnal Sosioteknologi, 18*(3), 509–516.

Jiang, Q., Zhang, Y., & Pian, W. (2022). Chatbot as an emergency exist: Mediated empathy for resilience via human-AI interaction during the COVID-19 pandemic. *Information Processing & Management, 59*(6), 103074. https://doi.org/10.1016/j.ipm.2022.103074

Khadpe, P., Krishna, R., Fei-Fei, L., Hancock, J. T., & Bernstein, M. S. (2020). Conceptual metaphors impact perceptions of human-AI collaboration. *Proceedings of the ACM on Human-Computer Interaction, 4*(CSCW2), 1–26.

Laestadius, L., Bishop, A., Gonzalez, M., Illenčík, D., & Campos-Castillo, C. (2022). Too human and not human enough: A grounded theory analysis of mental health harms from emotional dependence on the social chatbot Replika. *New Media & Society*, 14614448221142008.

Maples, B., Cerit, M., Vishwanath, A., & Pea, R. (2024). Loneliness and suicide mitigation for students using GPT3-enabled chatbots. *NPJ Mental Health Research, 3*(1), 4.

Mayer, J. D., & Salovey, P. (1995). Emotional intelligence and the construction and regulation of feelings. *Applied and Preventive Psychology, 4*(3), 197–208.

Mensio, M., Rizzo, G., & Morisio, M. (2018). The rise of emotion-aware conversational agents: threats in digital emotions. *In Companion Proceedings of the The Web Conference 2018* (pp. 1541–1544). https://doi.org/10.1145/3184558.3191607

Natale, S. (2019). If software is narrative: Joseph Weizenbaum, artificial intelligence and the biographies of ELIZA. *New Media & Society, 21*(3), 712–728.

Pink, S., & Leder Mackley, K. (2013). Saturated and situated: Expanding the meaning of media in the routines of everyday life. *Media, Culture & Society, 35*(6), 677–691. https://doi.org/10.1177/0163443713491298

Skjuve, M., Følstad, A., Fostervold, K. I., & Brandtzaeg, P. B. (2021). My chatbot companion—A study of human-chatbot relationships. *International Journal of Human-Computer Studies, 149*, 102601.

Sulaiman, S., Mansor, M., Wahid, R. A., & Azhar, N. A. A. N. (2022). Anxiety assistance mobile apps chatbot using cognitive behavioural therapy. *International Journal of Artificial Intelligence, 9*(1), 17–23.

Ta, V., Griffith, C., Boatfield, C., Wang, X., Civitello, M., Bader, H., DeCero, E., & Loggarakis, A. (2020). User experiences of social support from companion chatbots in everyday contexts: Thematic analysis. *J Med Internet Res, 22*(3), e16235. https://doi.org/10.2196/16235

Trothen, T. J. (2022). Replika: Spiritual enhancement technology? *Religions, 13*(4), 275.

Weizenbaum, J. (1976). *Computer power and human reason: From judgment to calculation.* W. H. Freeman & Co.

Weizenbaum, J., & Wendt, G. (2015). *Islands in the cyberstream: Seeking havens of reason in a programmed society.* Litwin Books.

Wibhowo, C., & Sanjaya, R. (2021). Virtual assistant to suicide prevention in individuals with borderline personality disorder. In *2021 International Conference on Computer & Information Sciences* (ICCOINS) (pp. 234–237). IEEE. https://doi.org/10.1109/ICCOINS49721.2021.9497160

Ziemer, K. S., & Korkmaz, G. (2017). Using text to predict psychological and physical health: A comparison of human raters and computerized text analysis. *Computers in Human Behaviour, 76*, 122–127.

CHAPTER 4

Developing a Smart Ecologies Approach to MHapp Research and Evaluation

Abstract In this chapter, we focus on a conceptually informed ecological approach to MHapp research and evaluation that addresses the role of automation. MHapps are part of an increasing integration of smart technologies in everyday life, which work through generating and capturing huge amounts of individual- and population-level data. The automation of MHapps means that support is not fixed to the specific locations of in-person support. Analytic approaches are needed that can capture the use of MHapps in real time in the everyday ecologies of individual users' lives. Drawing on the concept of the *smartness mandate* (Halpern & Mitchell, 2022) and the notion of *individuation* (Simondon & Adkins, 2020), we argue for a *smart ecologies* approach that captures the ways that the impacts of MHapps on individuals' mental health operate through multi-layered temporal and spatial dimensions, rather than the manifestation of factors (e.g. biological, psychological, social) that interact at the level of individual bodies to *cause* mental ill-health. We discuss the value of evaluation methods designed to gather 'real-world/real-time' data (e.g Ecological Momentary Assessment) and develop these through a smart ecologies approach conceptually informed by the notion of individuation.

Keywords Ecologies • Individuation • Smartness • Evaluation

L. Goodings et al., *Understanding Mental Health Apps*, Palgrave Studies in Cyberpsychology,
https://doi.org/10.1007/978-3-031-53911-4_4

The Ecologies of MHapps

This chapter focuses on articulating a conceptual approach to addressing the impact of mental health apps through capturing the *smart* and *affective* operation of ecologies of mental health apps. The drive for technologies to be *smart* continues apace, with many mental health apps being designed with layers of automation in their operation. The *smartness* of technologies therefore creates new kinds of relationships with our everyday environments. As detailed in Chaps. 1 and 2, affect studies offers conceptual insight for the study of mental health as operating through multiple relations between psychological, social, and material forces, which makes it difficult to reduce an individual's mental health experience to a singular factor, such as a biochemical irregularity in the brain. An approach that can fully capture the internal and external forces that shape individual experience is needed.

MHapps are part of the move to make societies *smarter* through the use of digital technologies driven by big data and automation. The *smartness mandate* (Halpern & Mitchell, 2022) argues that smartness works through identifying relations between individuals and population-data, a process subject to a significant acceleration due to the digitization of society. As such, a technology such as a MHapp is not only operating in terms of being designed to positively affect an individual's mental health but is part of a more complex ecology operating as the systematic relating of population-level data to individual user data. The data practices that are enabled by smart technologies such as MHapps can be thought to operate through creative new forms of value generation from the relationship of user data and population-level data. This is a point identified by Zuboff (2019) in terms of *surplus* value. With MHapps, this can be thought of as the data that is collected when users interact with the app, such as patterns of use, responses, reviews, etc. This may well be anonymized but is collected by smart technologies as part of their 'learning' process to become even smarter. This is the key premise upon which smart technologies operate, they are designed to appeal due to their technological prowess, and yet they are reliant on being used to become even 'smarter'. In a sense, they can be thought of as always in *beta* mode. Without the ability to constantly generate new data, their 'smartness' is limited.

Halpern and Mitchell's smartness mandate is that "all social processes become smart" (2022, p. 219). This chapter takes this idea to consider what it means for technologies for mental health support to become smart through automation. In the case of MHapps, we can think of surplus value being generated that allows for the realization of capital in terms of commercial and economic gain for developers. It is noteworthy that a significant proportion of MHapps is developed by private companies, at least initially, which can be sold to public health services. This is part of what Halpern and Mitchell (2022) refer to as an *epistemology of derivation*, namely an approach to understanding 'smartness' as fundamentally based on operating derivatively, which "underpins our contemporary lives" (p. 161). The derivative power of smart technologies to generate value, which is primarily monetized, requires critical approaches driven by desires to ensure smart technologies work towards, rather than against, equity. This is an important point in relation to MHapps, as to date, little is known in terms of the equity impacts of their use (Ramos et al., 2021).

In tracing the impact of smartness in relation to MHapps, it is important to conceptualize MHapp use as experienced in and through ecologies of relational processes involving bodies, technologies, and spaces. This is because smartness works through automating support, and therefore, it is not bound to the physical locations of in-person support (e.g. doctor-patient consultation). Automated support can be provided anywhere and at any time. The smart ecologies of MHapps therefore involve the generation of data through temporalities of everyday use, of which the app is one dimension. This is why it is important for the unit of analysis to extend beyond the individual user-MHapp relations. There are multiple dimensions at work in the everyday operation of MHapps, which exist at the interconnection of several body-technology-environments systems. These include the aforementioned individual user data and population-level data interaction; the temporal interactions with existing habits along with the creation of new habitual practices; as well as the spatial interactions in terms of the locational settings of MHapp use. These can be considered to co-constitute the ecologies of MHapps. Smartness points to distributed knowledge, and we argue that a conceptual approach is needed to understand how automated support operates in a distributed way across the environments that constitute individuals' everyday lives.

There has been limited focus on how smart technologies create new modes of orienting to our environments in relation to mental health. This chapter draws conceptual attention to the potential transformations of MHapps as smart technologies to transform users' relationships with their environments. Understanding the nature of these changes is central for capturing and identifying the impact of MHapps on users' mental health.

As noted in Chaps. 1 and 2, mental health is not solely an *internal* process, but it is shaped by a range of dimensions, which range from biochemical activity in the brain to the socio-material nature of the relationships with our everyday environments. As previously noted, clinical and neuroscientific research focused directly on the biochemical end of the spectrum of influence, with applied social research attending to the socio-material end of the spectrum. It is the impact of MHapps as key *agents* in the operation of users' mental health, constituted by a range of relations between bodies and ecologies that is the focus of this chapter.

Focusing on MHapps as smart technologies contributes to the growing body of research across the social sciences concerned with conceptualizing experiences of mental ill-health as operating through a network of social, material, and psychological relations (Duff, 2012; Reavey et al., 2019; Tucker & Goodings, 2014). This includes focusing on the affordances of specific settings on mental health (e.g. community and/or in-patient services) and understanding experiences of mental health as operating as multi-layered temporal and spatial forms. A socio-technical approach therefore needs to account for the distributed range of factors that can manifest as people's mental health experiences. Given the rise in prevalence of digital technologies in mental health support, there is a need to address their role as social and material agents in the constitution and operation of mental health.

The ecological approach in this chapter is a socio-technical one in terms of framing the impact of MHapps as new technologies of mental health support. Key here is analyzing what kinds of new relations with our everyday environments MHapps have the potential to create for users. Such relations do not manifest in a fixed manner but are subject to flexing in line with changing spatio-temporal forms. Indeed, experiences of mental health can be conceptualized *as* operating *as* spatial and temporal relations, rather than be considered as shaped by spatio-temporal practices existing *outside* of experience (Tucker & Lavis, 2019). In doing so, our approach to analyzing the *smartness* of MHapps is to conceptualize smartness as creating new spatio-temporalities that operate as relations with our everyday environments which manifest as mental health experiences. Furthermore, we argue for the need for approaches that can capture the fluidity and multi-dimensionality of the distributed operation of ecologies of MHapps. This is in recognition of the potential for our everyday environments to be ever-changing, hence the need to address the impact of MHapps in temporal as well as spatial terms. The concept of *smartness* captures this in terms of framing the operation of MHapps as experienced in relation to the fluid dynamics of changing environments. This extends nascent work emerging in the form of *critical ecological analysis* of youth mental health (Williams & Pykett, 2022). This chapter develops a specific focus on the *smartness* of mental health apps through articulating an approach to analyzing the impact of mental health apps that captures "how distress is shaped and mediated by technologies" (Williams & Pykett, 2022, p. 2), with the technologies in question being mental health apps. We are not presenting empirical analysis, but rather a conceptually informed approach to addressing the impacts of mental health apps that can inform future empirical studies. Part of this approach is to orient toward what apps *do*, rather than through a lens of *do they work* (Williams & Pykett, 2022). It is the latter that drives clinical research, but we argue that significant insight can be gained through addressing the former.

The notion of smartness speaks to the ways that mental health apps involve degrees of autonomy and agency in how they mediate people's mental health. Hence, MHapps come to affect the relations people have with their mental health, which is consequently framed not only at a biological level but also in terms of a broader set of social and technical relations, which come to constitute ecologies of mental health. This involves considering the affective operation of mental health app ecologies.

Atmospheres and Individuations

In Chaps. 1 and 2, we argued for the need to capture the *felt experience* of using apps to understand their impact. This means expanding the unit of analysis to include the setting/s of use, with affect studies pointing to the importance of attending to the broader network of relations in and through which individual and social life operates. In Chap. 2 we discussed how the concept of *atmosphere* can help to capture the extended affective operation of experience, showing how atmospheres operate as forms of potentialized affects that shape individual embodied experience. This is valuable as it allows for an approach that does not rely solely on the biological dimensions of mental health, but also the external social dimensions, not all of which may be actualized in any given situation or setting. This has been a major contribution of the concept of atmosphere to affect studies, part of the key argument that affect is not merely a supplement to cognition but rather plays an operational role in all dimensions of experience. To understand experience, one needs to understand affect. In this chapter, we extend the conceptual discussion of affective atmospheres through the notion of ***individuation*** in the philosophy of Gilbert Simondon. Individuation offers a complementary extended/distributed unit of analysis by placing emphasis on the conditions in and through which individual experiences and events actualize. Instead of starting with the experience/event itself and working ***backwards*** to understand its constitution, Simondon's notion of individuation starts with the wider context, or ***milieu*** in and through which the experience/event operates as a singularity from a broader set of potential experiences/events. The specifics of any given singularity cannot be known in advance and need to be analyzed as individuations. The notion of individuation offers a more explicit temporal focus than the spatial emphasis of atmospheres.

Simondon uses the example of crystallization to illustrate how individuation operates. The process of a crystal forming from a supersaturated solution operates through the solution ***having*** the potential for crystallization. As such, the solution can be considered as potentialized for the development of crystals. An individuation of a crystal is a process of singularity from a broader ecology (which Simondon names a ***milieu***) of potentialized energy. The crystal does not emerge and operate through the realization of a form/blueprint inherent to it, but rather its existence is understood in relation to the supersaturated solution as a milieu of potentialized energy. Its existence is not pre-determined in terms of being inevitable, but rather will only actualize given a certain set of conditions. This exemplifies how individuation works for Simondon. Analyzing a single individuation involves identifying the wider ecology *from* which it is actualized, and the conditions through which it operates. The environments of people's everyday lives are therefore considered as potentialized forms of energy, from which individual experiences actualize as singularities. The specifics of an individual experience cannot be fully known in advance, but rather need to be analyzed as spatio-temporal events. Any stability they show in terms of enduring in the form of a perceivable singularity (e.g. an individual body) needs to be analyzed in terms of the conditions of its persistence, not taken as being due to an inherent and stable form of identity.

The example of crystallization is an example of individuation in relation to non-living substances. Simondon also refers to forms of psychical individuation, in which emotion and affect play a primary role. This extends the discussion of affect in Chaps. 1 and 2, in relation to capturing the operation of affect in shaping, and being shaped by, a distributed set of socio-material relations, through which individual experiences are constituted and operate. The value of this for our analysis is demonstrating that the impact of MHapps, which is fundamentally premised as an *emotional* impact, is not solely about emotion affected solely by the relationship between a MHapp and an individual body, but rather as part of a broader understanding of the emotional life of a MHapp user. Emotion and affect are primary modes of relating that constitute an individuals' relationships with their everyday ecologies. This means that emotion in the form of an individual's mental health status cannot be 'ring fenced' from a broader emotional ecology emerging through a range of affective energies and forces. These are temporal and spatial, and complex. Hence the need for approaches that can capture this complexity.

We argue for approaches that extend beyond the strict relational approach that dominates clinical evaluation models, which frame the impacts of forms of mental health support in a strict intervention-effect variable model (Cromby et al., 2013). Such models have a clarity, but one that potentially comes at the cost of not capturing the broader set of relations that shape mental health experiences. What clinical interventionist models gain in methodological clarity, they lose in explanatory power. We argue for an ecological approach that can offer important explanatory power, which requires a degree of methodological complexity.

Evaluating the Impact of MHapps

Evaluations of mental health treatments typically take an individualized approach in terms of measuring whether the intervention has had a positive impact on a person's mental health. Such evaluations work in terms of operationalizing mental health in the form of a specific scale or measurement, e.g. in relation to depression, anxiety, and then gather pre and post-intervention measures at specific time points, with any change attributed to the intervention under focus (Cromby et al., 2013). Clinical evaluations can also include qualitative data collection in the form of interviews, visual materials, etc. Qualitative data collection often requires people to reflect on their experiences post-hoc, with reflections forming the material for analysis. Methodologies have emerged that aim to capture data in real time including temporal changes. These are broadly framed as forms of ecological momentary assessment (EMA) that claim to capture evaluation data 'in the field'. EMA was developed to provide a clinical evaluation method that can overcome some of the issues with evaluation methods based on post-intervention recall, e.g. accuracy (Stone et al., 2023). In this section, we will explore what kind of ecological approach EMA offers and what it can (and cannot) contribute to a *smart ecologies* approach.

Shiffman et al. (2008) define EMA as involving "repeated sampling of subjects' current behaviours and experiences in real time, in subjects' natural environments" (p. 1). In doing so EMA aims to "minimise recall bias, maximise ecological validity, and allow study of micro processes that influence behaviour in real-world contexts" (p. 1). One of the reasons that EMA is deemed valuable is that it can capture data regarding people's mental health *where and when* it is experienced, i.e. in the environments that constitute their everyday lives. EMA is perceived to provide data that are *close in time and space* to the experience under focus (e.g. individuals' feelings of depression, anxiety). It is this closeness that is reported as a major advantage of EMA, as the further data collection is from the time and space of the behavior/activity/experience it relates to, the less valid it is considered (Moskowitz & Young, 2006).

It is important to note that EMA is not a single methodological approach but rather provides a framework for evaluations seeking to collect data relating to behavior and experience at different time points, settings, and in real time. Any evaluation following the principles of EMA will need to be designed in relation to its aims and objectives. EMA has been used in relation to a wide range of clinical diagnoses, including "addictive disorders, eating disorders, anxiety disorders, depression, bipolar disorder, schizophrenia, sexual dysfunction, and ADHD" (Shiffman et al., 2008, p. 6). The use of digital technologies in EMA has been popular, as they can provide reminders and prompts for individuals to report and record their data. In the past, devices such as pagers were used, through to smart watches and devices (e.g. Fitbits), some of which can collect data automatically.

EMA has been considered as the "gold standard for measuring experience" in clinical research (Stone et al., 2023, p. 123). This does not mean that issues have not been raised with EMA as a methodology. These largely concern the control of variables under focus in clinical and behavioral research. For instance, ensuring that when participants report of the desired time frame (i.e. experience in the moment) when completing EMA prompts, or are they reporting on a more extended time frame (e.g. the previous few hours)? How does a researcher know whether participants interpret the questions in EMA as designed? These are two of several issues raised by Stone et al. (2023) in a recent review of EMA research.

They offer some suggestions as to how to overcome these challenges, including the use of cognitive interviews. Moreover, their aim is to stimulate discussion and reflection on current EMA research methodologies, with the aim of strengthening their use and validity in future research (Stone et al., 2023).

It is our view that the principles of EMA approaches are valuable and speak to our aim for a smart ecologies approach to MHapp research. The focus on 'real time and real world' data collection offers much in terms of gaining important insight regarding the impact of MHapps on mental health. However, we note that EMA approaches to date have been undertaken mostly in clinical research, with an emphasis on experimental research evaluations, which collect quantifiable and measurable data. We argue that this is limiting in terms of the range of experiential data that can be collected. In addition, it would be valuable to collect qualitative data, textual and visual, which can capture rich insight regarding the ways that MHapps operate and impact on people's lives in terms of being a key actor in the ecologies that constitute their everyday lives. We argue for an expanded sense of what data is valuable in relation to the ecologies of everyday life. For instance, diaries (written, audio, video); physiological data (heart rate, daily activity levels, sleep-related); behavioral data (exercise); general activity data (e.g. work, leisure time).

One of the key lessons for an ecological approach to MHapps is the idea that their impact on experiences of mental ill-health is not reducible in entirety to the specific intervention or content they provide, e.g. mindfulness, CBT. Rather, they become an object in and through which users interact with their everyday environment. This is fundamentally relational and processual, as our encounters and interactions with our environments are subject to temporal change. This is an advantage of models of evaluation such as EMA, as they can capture change over time, and do not rely on retrospective reports at fixed time points.

Toward a Smart Ecologies Approach

What would a smart ecologies evaluative model look like in practice? Grounding it in the principles of EMA is a good starting point. The regular reporting and recording of evaluative data 'in real time' provides important *temporal* data for an ecological approach. What it does not by definition provide is data that capture the expanded and distributed experience of MHapp use in spatial terms. This requires designing forms of data collection that directly capture the smart ecologies of use and experience. The use of visual methodologies is of value here. For instance, asking participants to record the settings of use of their MHApp use. This could include photos of the places they tend to use their MHApp, or drawings/pictures. Short video clips could also be included. These can easily be collected with smartphones. These could be supplemented by short written, audio, visual narratives about how the person is feeling at moments of data collection. Combining visual data and participants reports of their emotions 'in real time' is a valuable way to collect rich data regarding their experiences of the smart ecologies of MHApp use. These could be supplemented with quantitative data in the form of regularly completing mental health questionnaires and/or collecting physiological data. This approach can empirically capture insight regarding the individuations of experiences of mental health, through emphasizing their operation as a network of relations that combine to form the context of an individual's mental health experience.

Existing MHapp evaluations have tended to focus on well-established and popular current apps, such as Woebot, Wysa, Headspace, etc. These include the use of AI (artificial intelligence) technologies in the form of conversational agents, otherwise known as "chatbots". These apps automate decisions about which types of psychological support might be most beneficial for a user, based on data derived from AI technology. This highlights the value of thinking about the application of a smart mandate in the development of apps, with Woebot being a key example. Woebot is a conversational relational agent that offers CBT-based support of a textual nature through conversations with a bot in an app. Woebot asks for information in a chat style (e.g. mood) and then offers skills, tools, and ways of supporting psychological issues as part of the interaction in the app. This communication is directed to the Woebot avatar and responses are set into an ongoing conversational style. Using Large Language Models (LLM), Woebot accesses deep learning algorithms to recognize, summarize, and generate content from very large data sets. Through this complex analysis of LLMs, Woebot continues to "learn" ways of understanding human intent and improving human-like appropriate responses. The support is delivered through the Woebot LIFE app and each conversation begins with the general enquiry about the user ("what's going on in your world right now?") and appreciation of their mood ("how are you feeling?"). After providing this information, the user is then directed to CBT-content or word-games that are designed to educate users on core CBT principles and other forms of support.

As with many other MHapps, existing evaluations of Woebot have typically been of a clinical nature, aiming to demonstrate its impact using RCTs. For example, Durden et al. (2023) undertook an 8-week intervention trial investigating the use of Woebot for the reduction of stress and burnout. Such evaluations focus directly on the relationship between the app as an intervention and the users' mental health, as measured through an existing psychological scale. The smart ecologies approach we offer in this chapter would extend this evaluative framework through a more detailed analysis of 'real time' relational impact through capturing multiple data points (e.g. daily over a two-month period) and situating use of the app in a network of relations (e.g. time of day, location). This facilitates a broader evaluative framework that captures the whole ecology of use. This can help to enrich understanding of the multiple dimensions that contribute to people's experiences of using MHapps. In relation to an app such as Woebot, a smart ecological approach could include analysis of specific aspects of the app. For instance, it could identify whether users engage with the CBT element at specific times of the day and/or locations. It may be that different ecologies feature for different aspects of the app. This would be interesting as it could identify the broader impacts of different parts of the app's provision, which would be very valuable to know, rather than homogenizing the app's impact.

A smart ecologies approach would therefore involve identifying and attending to the specifics of the MHapps under evaluation, through an analysis that identifies the network of relations between specific functions and activities of MHapps and their ecologies. Multiple ecologies can exist in relation to one MHapp. Designing a smart ecological evaluation of a MHapp would follow a process of understanding how the app functions and its desired effect. Mapping the different activities of the app would provide a framework for the evaluative framework, as it will identify which functions' data need to be collected about users' engagement with the app. Furthermore, operationalizing the conceptualization of MHapp use as *individuations* draws attention to the temporalities of MHapp smart ecologies, meaning that evaluation frameworks need to attend to the temporal character of the impacts of MHapps. Their affects on users' mental health cannot be reduced to a relationship between the app and an individual's mental health state at a given moment, and not necessarily as a stable affect. As detailed in earlier chapters, affects are mobile and mutable, shaped by, and shaping of, relational processes between multi-dimensional ecologies that constitute individual and social life. The notion of individuation helps to conceptualize this operation, and hence the need for evaluation models to incorporate temporal analysis.

The MHapp example used in this chapter is Woebot, but the approach would apply to any MHapp, including popular ones such as Wysa, Headspace, etc. The smart ecologies approach can speak to approaches drawing on science and technology studies, and cultural studies, that offer new methods for fine grained analysis of "an apps intended purpose, embedded cultural meanings, and implied users and uses" (Light et al., 2018, p. 881). For instance, the *walkthrough* method to the study of apps, which is an ethnographic approach for researchers to analyze, step by step, the intended design of each part of an app (e.g. registration, daily use, etc.) and the cultural references recruited in its design. This can then provide insight regarding potential user experience. The walkthrough method was designed for use with researchers rather than users and is focused on the internal workings of apps, rather than the broader ecology of their use. We recognize potential scope for a smart ecologies approach that incorporates new methods such as the walkthrough method to gather rich data on the technical design of the multiple dimensions of MHapps, along with individual user experience, and how these come together as the relational operation of individuation.

References

Cromby, J., Harper, D., & Reavey, P. (2013). *Psychology, mental health and distress*. Palgrave Macmillan.

Duff, C. (2012). Exploring the role of 'enabling places' in promoting recovery from mental illness: A qualitative test of a relational model. *Health & Place, 18*(6), 1388–1395. https://doi.org/10.1016/j.healthplace.2012.07.003

Durden, E., Pirner, M. C., Rapoport, S. J., Williams, A., Robinson, A., & Forman-Hoffman, V. L. (2023). Changes in stress, burnout, and resilience associated with an 8-week intervention with relational agent 'Woebot'. *Internet Interventions, 33*, 100637. https://doi.org/10.1016/j.invent.2023.100637

Halpern, O., & Mitchell, R. (2022). *The smartness mandate*. MIT Press.

Light, B., Burgess, J., & Duguay, S. (2018). The walkthrough method: An approach to the study of apps. *New Media & Society, 20*(3), 881–900. https://doi.org/10.1177/1461444816675438

Moskowitz, D. S., & Young, S. N. (2006). Ecological momentary assessment: What it is and why it is a method of the future in clinical psychopharmacology. *The Journal of Psychiatry & Neuroscience, 31*, 13–20. https://doi.org/10.1186/1471-2369-15-29

Ramos, G., Ponting, C., Labao, J. P., & Sobowale, K. (2021). Considerations of diversity, equity, and inclusion in mental health apps: A scoping review of evaluation frameworks. *Behaviour Research and Therapy, 147*, 103990. https://doi.org/10.1016/j.brat.2021.103990

Reavey, P., Brown, S. D., Kanyeredzi, A., McGrath, L., & Tucker, I. (2019). Agents and spectres: Life-space on a medium secure forensic psychiatric unit. *Social Science & Medicine, 220*, 273–282. https://doi.org/10.1016/j.socscimed.2018.11.012

Shiffman, S., Stone, A. A., & Hufford, M. R. (2008). Ecological momentary assessment. *Annual Review of Clinical Psychology, 4*(1), 1–32. https://doi.org/10.1146/annurev.clinpsy.3.022806.091415

Simondon, G., & Adkins, T. (2020). *Individuation in light of notions of form and information*. University of Minnesota Press.

Stone, A. A., Schneider, S., & Smyth, J. M. (2023). Evaluation of pressing issues in ecological momentary assessment. *Annual Review of Clinical Psychology, 19*(1), 107–131. https://doi.org/10.1146/annurev-clinpsy-080921-083128

Tucker, I. M., & Goodings, L. (2014). Sensing bodies and digitally mediated distress serres, simondon, and social media. *Senses and Society, 9*(1). https://doi.org/10.2752/174589314X13834112761047

Tucker, I. M., & Lavis, A. (2019). Temporalities of mental distress: Digital immediacy and the meaning of 'crisis' in online support. *Sociology of Health & Illness, 41*(S1), 132–146. https://doi.org/10.1111/1467-9566.12943

Williams, J. E., & Pykett, J. (2022). Mental health monitoring apps for depression and anxiety in children and young people: A scoping review and critical ecological analysis. *Social Science & Medicine*, 297. https://doi.org/10.1016/j.socscimed.2022.114802

Zuboff, S. (2019). *The age of surveillance capitalism: The fight for a human future at the new frontier of power*. Profile Books.

CHAPTER 5

Moving Forward with MHapps

Abstract This book has sought to problematize a purely clinical approach for exploring MHapps and has adopted the use of a vital materialist perspective for studying the sociocultural dimensions of MHapps. In looking at applied examples in the previous chapters, we have outlined some of the alternative ways of studying MHapps and started to explore the complex ways that affect flows through these spaces. In this final chapter, we aim to draw together some practical conclusions and identify the main areas of interest for an applied psychosocial perspective of MHapps. This perspective resists an individual, internal logic that would seek to locate any change from using an app in a discrete set of psychological phenomena. Instead, we have been interested in the capacity for the body to be affected and to affect others. This focuses on the potential (or restrictions) for movement and the ways that bodies feel empowered to move in the context of the available atmospheres and the assemblage of the relations therein.

Keywords Algorithms • Atmospheres • Ecologies • Hope • Mental health • Momentary assessment • Shared emotion

L. Goodings et al., *Understanding Mental Health Apps*, Palgrave Studies in Cyberpsychology,
https://doi.org/10.1007/978-3-031-53911-4_5

Affective Life in MHapps

Analyzing the experience of MHapps involves understanding the relationships people have with themselves and others, and how these relationships are constituted through the datafication of everyday life of living with MHapps. An applied psychosocial approach is interested in the relational processes that emerge from the coming together of multiple bodies in space, the actions therein, and the subsequent impact on experience. In engaging with MHapps, users are regularly faced with the issue of how to manage the attempts of trying to act into the app to create meaning, while also accepting that this may result in unexpected changes because of these actions. Whether a user is self-tracking one's mood via Daylio, building a relationship with a Replika, or asking Woebot for help with feelings of anxiety, there is one thing that is shared by all these actions: they seek to continue positive relations that enable future potentials to act and be acted upon in multiple ways. "Affects", Anderson argues, move between people in processes of intersubjective transmission to *make a space for hope*" (2006, p. 744). This "space for hope" is characteristic of the actions in MHapps in which there is a continuous set of actions and activities that are part of the everyday engagement with the space. Therefore, feeling hopeful is an emergent affective property of the continuation of moving and interacting within an app. Hopefulness in MHapps emerges from the perpetual state of "on-ness" (Pink & Leder Mackley, 2013) that keeps the affective space-time of an app alive with movement and affords future potentials for self-discovery. In discussing the role of vital memorial practices and the anticipatory feeling of affect, Brown and Reavey argue:

> We do not just think the past: we are touched by it affectively. The material and cognitive affordances of invariant assemblies of relations lure us into feelings about past persons and events that can be both ambiguous and challenging ... we have defined affect as the 'feeling of affordance', the felt sense of the possible (what we can do and what can be done to us) that arises from our engagement with assemblies of relations. (2015, p. 220)

Collecting MHapp data does not directly contribute to *feeling better* but is imbued with, as Brown and Reavey (2015) argue, a "felt sense" of the invariant ability to affect or be affected. MHapp users get a sense of the possible potential for affectivity through the anticipatory ways that they can move and act in an app. This *feeling* is indeterminate given that there is no direct relationship between what we think and feel and what will come to happen. But it leaves a residual feeling, a sense of the possible. Collecting data on their mood does not make a MHapp user feel better, but it opens the door to being affected. As such, there are certain moments that punctuate this flow of experience and provide a snapshot of the current capacity to act, followed by a feeling of how we are situated in the world. To emphasize this point, Brown and Reavey (2015) use the children's game of musical chairs as an example: when each child is moving around the chairs everything is fine, but at the moment the music stops there is a cause for concern, there is a need to *take stock* of the current position in relation to the other players and find a way to move to a space that will allow the game to continue, in this case, to find a free chair. In MHapps, there are many instances when the music stops (a new piece of data arrives, someone new enters the atmosphere) and there is a pause in how we are relating to others, resulting in a felt sense of how we belong in the world. It is at this moment that we must take ownership of our feelings and make sense of our future capacity to act and in relation to other bodies.

Continually adding information to MHapps and re-narrativizing information from an app means that users are continually striving to create a space for hope in the future. This drive for the sense of the possible might also mean that, for many, it makes sense to keep the game alive by continually adding or changing something in the app and thus avoiding the need to pause and 'take ownership' of the current affective position. This concept aligns with Spinoza's early reading of affect which defines joy (or hope in this case) as the passage from lesser to greater perfection and sadness as the reverse, from greater to lesser perfection (Gatens & Lloyd, 2002). Therefore, users are locked in an ever-changing set of affective atmospheres in which it is easier to keep moving and interacting. This brings us to thinking about the temporal aspects of MHapp usage in the next section.

(Re)framing MHapps in Space and Time

In the discussion of MHapps in this book, we have often spoken of the way that affect emerges from a specific space that shapes (and is shaped by) how bodies come together in apps. The discussion of the spatial elements of the interaction has been (hopefully!) well-documented in this book, but we wanted to take a moment to further tease-out the unique features of the way that *time* functions as a vital aspect of the affective experience of moving through MHapps. In conducting a clinical review of an app, time is presented as a variable which needs to be experimentally *controlled* and *contained*. But what if we wanted to take a more complex view of time? One where we wanted to accept the temporal aspects of experience, as opposed to removing these issues in the pursuit of a scientific appreciation of apps? In fact, if we consider the ways that people have been shown to use apps so far in this book, be that in terms of the direct materials of the app or reviewing the data produced by the app, these impacts never seem to be in a linear fashion: users jump to particular content, swipe over to a different section of the app, look at some of their information from a previous use, and then slip back into a video they know that they enjoy. As a result, their usage is characterized by an ongoing switching, overlapping, and mutual shaping of simulation and experience. This chapter will now explore some applied examples of this issue, taking further examples from the self-tracking data from Chap. 2 and beginning with an example of how the concept of AI is discussed by one of the participants. In the following example, the discussion centers around the incorporation of AI technologies into a mediation and mindfulness app:

Example 5.1
I think it just depends on what way it's used and but also I feel like if it's used more and more than that takes away some of the natural side of things and then like what are human beings except for spontaneous and natural, you know and and quirky. In the same way that I was saying about you don't like to be told how you feel. It's like AI is assuming how you are that day.

Example 5.1 shows a common response about any future uses of AI technologies being used to 'predict' how they are feeling or provide ways of anticipating a particular emotional state in the future. All participants expressed concern about how the AI technologies would function in the future, with increased presence of AI. In this context, time feels stretched and unknown (as the changes to AI are hidden to the user), but where the presence of these changes looms large over the proceedings. As the participant states, they are unsure how this app will continue to feel "natural", and how they are already aware they will take issue with the app telling them exactly how to feel. What is striking about the way that this story is being told is the impact of the sense of different affective forces (AI in the future) and the way that this is relationally enacted. In this case, time becomes relevant in terms of an indeterminate character through which the participant envisages a changing relationship with the self, wherein interactions with AI bodies' results are constructed as being characterized by an inability to feel "natural" and "spontaneous". Notice the way that the affective aspects of this situation are not felt in terms of a singular time-point or a singular subject. The concern about AI inclusion in the use of MHapps is felt in terms of a past, present, and future affective aspects of these issues. Next, we look at another example of how time is conceptualized in the use of MHapps. This extract is taken from a diary entry of one of the participants who documented their use of the Feeling Good app (positive mindset and typically intended for reducing stress and anxiety). This diary entry was recorded while they were using the app and was directed at identifying how useful they were finding the app:

Example 5.2
In a few words the app is very calming and reassuring which I find useful because I'm quite an anxious person and I stress myself out with overthinking.

It's like when my mind is going a million miles an hour with all the things I must do and the worries I have and it's all so loud, taking the time to listen to the audio just makes everything quiet again.

Example 5.2 shows how accessing the atmosphere in the app affords a way of attending to their psychological state (where their "mind is going a million miles an hour"). And while this might typically be identified in terms of the unique spatial features of the app, the temporal aspects of this experience are also pivotal in the affective dimensions of this process. Coleman (2018) argues that within the ongoing patterns of digital usage a temporal present emerges that focuses on "the now" in the present, but also speaks to the ongoing, open-ended, and vibrant possibilities in the future. Coleman describes "*infra*-structures of feeling" as a way of accounting for the systems and linkages via which the affectivity of the present is encountered and experienced (Coleman, 2020, 2022). Following this view, MHapps also seem to hold-together a range of competing hopes and desires in the present, which are also characterized by a sense of the temporary and changing aspects of the experience. Example 5.2 shows the experience of using the app in a stressful situation and how this is laden with feelings of movement and change, where the participant states that using the app enables them to transition from a negative set of feelings to a moment where the app "makes everything quiet again". This feels 'alive' with temporal possibility and performs the experience of using the app with a sense of vitality and movement—it provides a way of structuring these feelings. The participant describes being able to see their mental health in terms of the potential for change, as moving from one state to another. This temporal aspect of the experience is important in the recollection of the event and is imbued with the desire to feel differently about their mental health. As with spatial attempts at acting in the atmosphere, temporal forms of affect also carry an invariant character, but the power is in the way the app affords a sense of past, present, and future forms of affects all bound-up in the way that app is being mediated in "the now" (see also Simmons et al., 2023). Therefore, even if the app does not show the exact desired performance of mental health in the present "now", via the inherent sense of movement that is invested in the app, the user is still able to feel optimistic about their psychological health in the future via the mediation of a future state of their health. The process is never complete and involves a temporal present that is alive to future possibilities for change.

Slater (2014) considers the way that any discussion of affective atmospheres typically obfuscates the temporal aspects of atmospheres, arguing that there is an over-focus on the spatial features of atmospheres. This perspective advocates discussion of the temporal-material unfolding of experience in affective atmospheres, in which timings are never "mono-temporal" or singular in character (Slater, 2014). For an appreciation of the temporal aspects of atmospheres to be possible, Slater acknowledges the need to accept Böhme's (2017) proposition to "liberate" the subject-object binary of atmospheres, recognizing that as there is no clearly bonded subject or "I" that is affected, as this affection cannot be located or situated at any singular moment in time. This is further shared in Brennan's (2004) view as atmospheres (although there are other critiques of this application) as neither being in the environment or in the person, providing a helpful way of *dis*-locating time and space. This appreciates the constant state of ongoing transformations and transitions that emerge from any atmosphere that are based on a particular arrangement of space *and* time. Brown et al. (2019) argue, "rather than say that atmospheres are *in* space or time, envelopment constitutes its own specific *space-time*" (p. 7). Therefore, atmospheres in MHapps are continually fluctuating and not bound to a moment in time of personal subjective experience, nor are they a temporal localization of the environmental presence of the world in the app itself. Alternatively, they are a product of the unique atmospheric space-time that has the potential to move, shape, and change us as we navigate the entangled bodies therein. The role of the atmospheres in apps will now be summarized.

Atmospheres and Shared Emotion in MHapps

Atmospheres are ephemeral, indeterminate totalities that are void of subject or object, but, as we have seen from the data in earlier chapters, atmospheres can "grip" a person and induce ways of feeling. The exploration of MHapps in this book has shown that affects can be felt in terms of a snapshot of the current status of psychological health and wellbeing, in which MHapp users are regularly confronted with a choice of whether to stop and take stock of their feelings or to keep the profile moving and changing by acting into the atmosphere. For this reason, it makes 'app' sense to have multiple possible avenues for keeping the body alive via a range of potential atmospheres. In Chap. 3, the update to the ERP function in Replika caused significant disruption in the way that users could maintain emotional connections with their Replikas. These changes resulted in the community of users taking to Reddit to describe these issues and a discussion formed around the collective impact of the updates that occurred in February 2023. For many, the changes meant that it was impossible to continue using their Replika as a source of psychological support, showing how affective processes are shaped by changes from non-human bodies and how atmospheres can be felt at a collective level. Trigg (2020, p. 3) recognizes the shared emotional aspects of atmospheres and explains how "the grasping of atmospheres through the lived experience of the body seldom takes place in isolation". Trigg argues that atmospheres function by generating a mutual awareness of others and by conjoining members of an atmosphere into a sense of integrative togetherness. In the discussion with participants, they regularly spoke of the ways that they expected others to act or how they would be worried about the implications of how a certain action might seem to others. Thus, the ERP updates generated a mutual sense of others in the experience and united the members in a sense of togetherness. This creates, as Trigg would argue, a force of cohesion between participants, and when there is then greater attunement to the atmosphere, there is then an enhanced sense of the cohesion with others. Meaning that:

> The advent of a hopeful atmosphere is something that belongs to us (as *our* hope) and to which we ourselves as supporters belong to it (as *our* atmosphere). Such an atmosphere serves not only as a force of momentum, but also as a force of cohesion between the participants. (Trigg, 2020, p. 6)

In being gripped by an atmosphere in an app and sensing the body through the affective changes is to feel the potential of that space: importantly, this allows for collective, shared feelings that connects with others via a community of others who connect with this experience. Furthermore, these actions contribute to a sense of a cohesion between a group of people that are jointly immersed in the practices of the atmosphere, in this case, the practice of self-tracking mental health via an app. At moments of heightened active attunement to the atmosphere (such as in dealing with a stressful situation), this is coupled with a sense of togetherness with others who are responding to mental health concerns via an app in a similar fashion.

Ecologies of Mental Health in Apps

Distress can take many forms, and MHapps are just one way of attending to psychological health and wellbeing. Digital technologies do not function in a psychological vacuum, and studying apps *before and after* any given usage does not account for the ways that affect transcends spatially and temporarily distributed encounters. Thinking about the spatio-temporal forms of atmospheres connects with other advances in critical ecological analysis and acts as a useful reminder of the need to situate apps as one entry point for engaging with our mental health. This requires a more *expanded* view of the way we relate to ourselves and other bodies than is available in a typical psychological assessment of apps, and via the medical model more generally. Turnbull et al. (2023) uses the term digital ecologies to describe the "human-nonhuman relations which favors situated understandings of digitisation as a material, affective and plural process" (p. 4). This shows a growing use of the term ecology to understand and describe the more-than-human environments in which MHApps are located. Turnbull et al. stresses the *plurality* of digital affective interactions that captures the experimental, *trial-and-error* type behavior through which people are constantly affecting (and being affected) in the process of acting into the digital world of apps. This might include taking a photograph related to a current experience, selecting an emoji to describe a current mood-state, telling a story about the data, or meeting with a mental health professional and mentioning how the app helps to reduce stress (or not). All these actions, taken together, forms a constantly evolving diverse ecology of overlapping human and non-human actions which requires a separation from the idea of apps as discreet "tools" (Williams & Pykett, 2022) for mental health and, instead, viewing these technologies as part of an extended, distributed form of technology that constitute a wider digital ecology of mental health (see also Fullagar, 2017). To that end, all the digital devices that have been discussed in these chapters are considered to be constituted in the everyday experience of engaging with our mental health: they are *part of*, not wholly responsible for, the ways that we encounter opportunities for transition and change, a process which is highly affectively charged.

The findings in this book are moving toward the type of understanding that stems from the ecological momentary analysis (EMA) approach presented in Chap. 4. Through the analysis of interviews, diary entries, and photographs, there is focus on *where* and *when* mental health is experienced and felt via an app. This shows how the EMA approach is valuable to researching MHapps as it unites with many principles of a vital materialist perspective given the focus on the relational, processual, and felt aspects of the automation of support through apps. This book has illustrated the benefit of using data 'in the field' to explore how people live in and through the digital material landscape of new technologies. It is important to note that EMA is not a single methodological approach but rather provides a framework for evaluations seeking to collect data relating to behavior and experience at different time points, settings, and in real time. One aspect of MHapps that will need to be further explored in the future is the role of the algorithm.

Algorithms in MHapps

In *Algorithmic Intimacy* (2023), Anthony Elliot discusses the rapid expansion of the "psychologization of contemporary social life" (p. 79) and considers the role of MHapps in the rising context of automated therapeutic technologies ("therapy tech"). Elliot considers the risks associated with linking AI with therapeutic culture and the potential for apps to be self-limiting as machines are largely "self-referential" and have the potential to dampen the personal and collective opportunities for advancement given the confines of the machine. Elliot recognizes how the digital revolution is transforming relationships and intimacy via the unprecedented power of predictive algorithms, highlighting the monopolizing influence of the algorithm in which the "machine knows best". As a result, according to Elliot, people habitually orient their feelings to non-human others and are routinely reminded to seek escape from engagement with others, which results in further cases of social isolation and loneliness. Yet, through a reordering of socio-technical practices, these outcomes can be avoided by seeking and encouraging people to act into algorithmic-driven spaces and question the life strategies that are unthinkingly and automatically enacted via machine intelligence.

Chapter 4 shows the complexity of feelings being generated through digital spaces in the emotional exchanges with AI technologies such as Replika. The role of AI and computer-generated forms of intimacy present challenges when the users become dependent on these relations and when they come to expect them to conform to human types of interaction. As the ERP updates showed, affect flowed differently through the space of interaction following these changes, as the Replika's ability to communicate was felt to have lost emotional capacity. The unintended consequence of these updates meant that users were unable to maintain relationships in the same way, given the emotional changes to their Replika. What this shows us is that these interactions *felt real* and that the affective atmospheres that are presented via these technologies constitute powerful spaces of self-knowledge and relational interaction. For many users, the update exposed the emotional changes to the Replika and were felt in terms of a significant inability to continue connecting with the technology. This resonated in terms of a mutual togetherness for those that could no longer maintain a relationship with their Replika. Therefore, it is necessary to continually revisit the extent to which people can align their thoughts, feelings, and actions with non-human others. For David Beer (2022), these tensions provide an opportunity to explore algorithmic thinking and illustrate the different types of automation that are unfolding in everyday life.

Virtual companion chatbots are likely to be pivotal in the future development of MHapps. The ability for these technologies to replicate the 'warmth' of human interaction is going to gather apace. However, the concern here, as Elliot suggests, is that this will reflect on human relation formation processes and will tend to encourage more narcissistic-type behaviors in the users, given the way that the technology is designed to promote a self-centered form of thinking. Instead, we need to find ways to continually explore the affective relationships and the way AI is contributing to the formation of feelings; ensuring that chatbot development is delivered in dialogue with potential users and in conjunction with the impacts on affective life of those who use Replika and other such services for psychological support is of crucial importance.

Conclusion: An Applied Psychosocial Perspective

In assessing new technologies like MHapps, research in psychology would typically seek to establish clinical evidence of the efficacy of such apps in terms of forms of distress (a reduction in anxiety, depression). While this has value in certain settings, this book has sought to extend the area of psychological thinking to include the social, cultural, and material dimensions of MHapp experience. Digitization of support and the ways that we can capture, monitor, and manage psychological health will continue apace. As with development of apps for physical health, the apps for psychological health are likely to continue to grow and find new avenues for measurement and collection, including biometric sensors and other ways of measuring the body. These developments will offer ways of classifying the body (e.g. via stress hormones) that may be read as indicators of psychological distress. This will be combined with the other types of information (e.g. self-report) and the ways of knowing the body will shift and change. This data will continue to be of commercial interest to large corporations and the balance of the perceived benefits of these apps versus the data mining practices/AI will shape new emotional and affective ways of understanding ourselves and others via an app. This will, in turn, require future analysis of the affective processes therein.

Throughout the book, we hope to have shown ways that the social, material, and psychological are intrinsically linked in the everyday use of apps. This has focused on the "lively" ways (Lupton, 2016) that data feature in the affective practices of engaging with apps for psychological support. This is a delicate business that requires living with atmospheres that are made-up of a constantly shifting set of relational assemblages that envelop from a unique space-time. The ability to feel the atmosphere will no doubt change as people gain further knowledge into data generation practices and there are further ways of visualizing the current bodies that are present in an atmosphere. This will lead to more opportunities for shared emotional responses and will allow for further study of the collective aspects of affective awareness in MHapps.

Digitization of psychological phenomena and the practices of self-tracking form the backbone of MHapp activity. The data that is generated through these processes is generated from the entangled interactions of bodies. This brings together a number of different data-bodies given that, as one participant stated, the data is the "mediator" for how they are feeling. This shows how data provides a bridge between body and technology in which there is a mutual shaping of body and experience. MHapps exist as a datafied space in which data is inextricably tied to the ability to feel about ourselves and others. Chapter 2 showed how self-tracking was found to be immersed in the ways that people can get a snapshot of how they are doing, as part of the ongoing practices of living with digital data and moving with (and responding to) the feelings that emerge from atmospheres in MHapps. It showed the ability to shape an atmosphere while simultaneously shaping (or being gripped) by atmospheres. These actions are always embodied and technologically mediated.

Chapters 3 and 4 illustrated new considerations for understanding the way that MHapps function in everyday life. For the users of Replika, behind-the-scenes changes to the emotional capacity of their AI companions sent a shockwave through the community and resulted in feelings of loss and separation for many. This shows just how much emotional support is flowing through these interactions and how the updates (or other technological interventions) are met with skepticism and suspicion from the users involved. These technologies have the power to serve as valuable therapeutic companions, but these powers are diminished through the interference from external sources. As with the discussion of the ELIZA chatbot, it was the users that first identified this technology as being particularly beneficial for psychological support. It is therefore important to continue the critical insight into the ways that people are mediating these technologies and the affective powers that are bestowed upon them. This work should also, however, remind users of the dangers of "breathing life into the machine", following Elliott's (2022) discussion of Replika, as it is important to encourage users to question the affective life strategies that are automatically introduced as commonplace, natural behavior.

This book has begun to gather evidence of the social, material, and cultural dimensions of MHapps, but this is only the start. Chapter 4 introduced a way of exploring the live experiences living with apps and purposefully directed attention to the relational, processual, and felt aspects of the automation of the available support through apps. This needs to go further to account for the spatial and temporal aspects of affective life in MHapps and explore how these technologies will continue to include other methods for data collection and link with other social technologies. This is the next stage for this research is to further comprehend the role of MHapps in the broader experiential environment of people's everyday lives.

References

Anderson, B. (2006). Becoming and being hopeful: Towards a theory of affect. *Environment and Planning D: Society and Space, 24*(5), 733–752.

Beer, D. (2022). *The tensions of algorithmic thinking: Automation, intelligence and the politics of knowing*. Policy Press.

Böhme, G. (2017). *The aesthetics of atmosphere*. Routledge.

Brennan, T. (2004). *The transmission of affect*. Cornell University Press.

Brown, S., & Reavey, P. (2015). *Vital memory and affect: Living with a difficult past*. Routledge.

Brown, S. D., Kanyeredzi, A., McGrath, L., Reavey, P., & Tucker, I. (2019). Affect theory and the concept of atmosphere. *Distinktion: Journal of Social Theory, 20*(1), 5–24.

Coleman, R. (2018). Theorizing the present: Digital media, pre-emergence and infra-structures of feeling. *Cultural Studies, 32*(4), 600–622.

Coleman, R. (2020). Making, managing and experiencing 'the now': Digital media and the compression and pacing of 'real-time'. *New Media & Society, 22*(9), 1680–1698.

Coleman, R. (2022). The presents of the present: Mindfulness, time and structures of feeling. *Distinktion: Journal of Social Theory, 23*(1), 131–148.

Elliott, A. (2022). *Algorithmic intimacy: The digital revolution in personal relationships*. John Wiley & Sons.

Fullagar, S. (2017). Post-qualitative inquiry and the new materialist turn: Implications for sport, health and physical culture research. *Qualitative Research in Sport, Exercise and Health, 9*(2), 247–257.

Gatens, M., & Lloyd, G. (2002). *Collective imaginings: Spinoza, past and present*. Routledge.

Lupton, D. (2016). Personal data practices in the age of lively data. *Digital Sociologies, 2016*, 335–350.

Pink, S., & Leder Mackley, K. (2013). Saturated and situated: Expanding the meaning of media in the routines of everyday life. *Media, Culture & Society, 35*(6), 677–691.

Simmons, N., Goodings, L., & Tucker, I. (2023). Experiences of using mental health Apps to support psychological health and wellbeing. *Journal of Applied Social Science*, *18*(1). https://doi.org/10.1177/19367244231196768

Slater, C. (2014). *Atmospheres of affect. In timing of affect: Epistemologies, aesthetics, politics*. Diaphanes.

Trigg, D. (2020). The role of atmosphere in shared emotion. *Emotion, Space and Society*, *35*, 100658.

Turnbull, J., Searle, A., Hartman Davies, O., Dodsworth, J., Chasseray-Peraldi, P., von Essen, E., & Anderson-Elliott, H. (2023). Digital ecologies: Materialities, encounters, governance. *Progress in Environmental Geography*, *2*(1–2), 3–32. https://doi.org/10.1177/27539687221145698

Index

L. Goodings et al., *Understanding Mental Health Apps*, Palgrave Studies in Cyberpsychology,
https://doi.org/10.1007/978-3-031-53911-4